CORE
PERFORMANCE
WOMEN

CORE
PERFORMANCE
WOMEN

Burn Fat and Build Lean Muscle

MARK VERSTEGEN
AND PETE WILLIAMS

AVERY
a member of Penguin Group (USA) Inc.
New York

Published by the Penguin Group

Penguin Group (USA) Inc., 375 Hudson Street, New York, New York 10014, USA

Penguin Group (Canada), 90 Eglinton Avenue East, Suite 700, Toronto, Ontario M4P 2Y3,

Canada (a division of Pearson Penguin Canada Inc.) · Penguin Books Ltd, 80 Strand, London WC2R 0RL, England

Penguin Ireland, 25 St Stephen's Green, Dublin 2, Ireland (a division of Penguin Books Ltd)

Penguin Group (Australia), 250 Camberwell Road, Camberwell, Victoria 3124, Australia

(a division of Pearson Australia Group Pty Ltd) · Penguin Books India Pvt Ltd,

11 Community Centre, Panchsheel Park, New Delhi–110 017, India

Penguin Group (NZ), 67 Apollo Drive, Rosedale, North Shore 0632, New Zealand

(a division of Pearson New Zealand Ltd) · Penguin Books (South Africa) (Pty) Ltd,

24 Sturdee Avenue, Rosebank, Johannesburg 2196, South Africa

Penguin Books Ltd, Registered Offices: 80 Strand, London WC2R 0RL, England

Most Avery books are available at special quantity discounts for bulk purchase for sales promotions, premiums, fund-raising, and educational needs. Special books or book excerpts also can be created to fit specific needs. For details, write Penguin Group (USA) Inc. Special Markets, 375 Hudson Street, New York, NY 10014.

Library of Congress Cataloging-in-Publication Data

Verstegen, Mark, date.

Core performance women : burn fat and build lean muscle / Mark Verstegen and Pete Williams.

p.   cm.

ISBN 978-1-58333-362-4

1. Endurance sports.   2. Physical fitness for women.   3. Exercise for women.   4. Nutrition.

I. Williams, Pete, date.   II. Title.

GV749.5.V49   2009   2009036194

613.7'045—dc22

Printed in the United States of America

1   3   5   7   9   10   8   6   4   2

BOOK DESIGN BY TANYA MAIBORODA

CONTENTS

CORE
PERFORMANCE
WOMEN

INTRODUCTION:
THE SPARTAN WOMAN

've always been fascinated by Spartan women. In ancient Greece they were strong and independent, enjoying a level of respect, power, and status unheard of in their time. They owned land, were literate, and were encouraged to exercise, even competing alongside men in athletic contests. With Spartan men often away at war, the women were in charge.

The image of the Spartan woman has been more visible recently, fueled by the popularity of the movie *300*. The actress Lena Headey stole the show with her powerful portrayal of Queen Gorgo, the wife of King Leonidas I.

According to legend, Gorgo once was asked why Spartan women were the only women in the world who could rule men. Her reply: "Because Spartan women are the only ones who can give birth to *real* men."

Today women rule the world. Perhaps not when it comes to political office, though that is changing all the time, but in all other aspects of life. Women control family budgets, take an ever-increasing role in corporate leadership, and make up 55 percent of college enrollments. They organize social networks for themselves, friends, and family members, and generally are viewed as the pillars of their families and social groups. And, of course, they deliver the miracle of life.

Yes, the image of the Spartan woman is alive and well and, if you're reading this book, I have no doubt you exhibit those qualities, much like my wife, mother, sisters, and countless family members, friends, and colleagues.

When Pete Williams and I were asked to write *Core Performance Women*, we were a little taken aback. After all, we possess Y chromosomes. Plus, we viewed our previous books as not solely for men.

If anything, women embrace the Core Performance system more quickly than men since women generally are more cognizant of issues such as hip stability, balance, energy levels, and the role of proper nutrition.

Ours is not a no-pain-no-gain program, but since women have a higher threshold for pain, they tend to be more persistent when it comes to meeting physical challenges. Judging by the feedback we've received from our previous books, women embraced the Core Performance system as much as, if not more than, men.

Then it dawned on us that none of our previous books—and perhaps none in this massive fitness-book genre—have been written with this Spartan woman in mind. Plenty of trees have fallen to produce quick-fix diet-and-exercise books to "tone up" and create the perfect bikini body, preferably in twelve weeks or less. But nobody has offered an integrated lifestyle system to support these remarkable people, who just happen to be women.

How could all of us in this industry have overlooked this group of high achievers? How could we have failed to provide a specific support system for the most overtaxed members of society?

It's not the first time this has happened. My career has focused on creating an industry that provides world-class support to elite athletes, enabling them to run faster and perform better, injury- and pain-free, for longer periods of time. That sounds like an obvious idea, but nobody had done it on a large scale previously.

In recent years we've extended this concept to top business executives. Thousands of employees count on their leaders for direction and guidance, especially during difficult times. Yet who is there to support the corporate leader, making sure she has a system in place to sustain her energy levels and overall well-being while preventing long term injury and ailments? Nobody, really. So we've provided that system for her.

And yet the vast majority of women still are unsupported, even though they fill the vital role of supporting and nurturing family and friends, typically more so than men, often in addition to playing a corporate leadership role. It's a job (or jobs) that's ever more pressure-packed in today's hectic, technology-based world where the obesity epidemic, economic crisis, and other concerns have converged to overwhelm even a Spartan woman.

When we talk about the human race or the "race involving humans," we know that women run a steeper grade than men. Marketers target girls as young as three with messages of how they must look and what they must eat. Boys spend their childhoods blissfully ignorant of such pressures (while getting away with everything, it seems).

Girls have more opportunities to play sports than they did just fifteen years ago but suffer ACL knee injuries at a far greater rate than boys, even though girls typically don't play football. Boys have it easier in the teenage years, with physical and hormonal changes that pale in comparison to dealing with the start of four decades of menstrual cycles.

The workplace, even with advances in recent decades, still is stacked in favor of men, who can wait until their forties or fifties to consider starting a family. Women feel more pressure to build careers quickly, at the expense of dating and social lives. Then, during a brief window in their middle to late thirties, they're expected to marry, have children, and shoulder most of the burden of dealing with toddlers—preferably while maintaining that high-paying career and reclaiming their pre-pregnancy bodies.

Women in their forties and fifties are held to the same physical standards as women half their age, while men grow "ruggedly handsome," gray, and fat. Sean Connery moved seamlessly from being James Bond to a bald sex symbol as a senior. It doesn't work that way for women, who also lose the ability to bear children long before men no longer can father them. About the time women are raising teenagers, still bearing most of that responsibility, their bodies revolt through menopause. Though women have a slight edge in life expectancy, their so-called golden years are more likely to include osteoporosis and related issues involving the loss of bone density.

Since the time of Queen Gorgo, the term *Spartan* has come to mean "marked by self-discipline or self-restraint." It means simple, frugal, courageous in the face of pain, danger, and adversity. We think of a Spartan lifestyle in terms of diet or home decor.

There's nothing wrong with most if not all of those traits, but the Core Performance system is not going to require you to exert excessive self-discipline, follow a diet of deprivation, or surrender the finer things in life. It *is* a simple system in that we boil things down to four pillars: the Core Fundamentals of Mindset, Nutrition, Movement, and Recovery, which you will design your entire life around.

Let me explain. If I offered you yet another diet-and-exercise regimen, it would be a struggle for you to sustain it. After all, you're overbooked as it is. How could you possibly carve out the time? And you'd be right. Instead, we're going to build your life around a system that will provide you with *more* time and energy by allowing you to perform better.

It's easy to get beaten down by our fast-paced culture, especially as many com- panies have stripped staffs and resources to the bone. (Talk about a Spartan existence!) People are working longer and harder for less money, handling job descriptions previously meant for two or three employees.

Against this backdrop, it's easy to abandon consistent exercise—or abstain from it altogether—and still feel like you'll come out ahead. So you grind harder, firm in the belief that you can outwork and outhustle anyone through sheer willpower.

Sooner or later your body will rebel, breaking down from illness or injury. It's a vicious downward spiral—the harder you work, the more run-down you become and the less energy you have. Nobody can keep up the pace forever unless they have a game plan to help.

At the moment, you're probably caught in reactive mode. Like someone trying to survive in a one-on-seven game of dodgeball, it's all you can do to handle everything thrown your way.

Let's say you're a young woman. You wake up in the morning after a short, restless sleep. You hustle out the door, grabbing "breakfast" on the go in the form of an expensive designer coffee and a bagel or muffin. At work you gulp down more coffee as you handle the jobs of two other people laid off because of the economy. Lunch, if you manage to find time, is takeout that offers little nutritional value. You're dragging by midafternoon, so you drink more caffeine and get a jolt of sugar from the vending machine. Still, you struggle to get as much work done as you'd like, so you stay until seven p.m., hoping to avoid the next downsizing. Because you want to maintain some semblance of a social life, you meet friends for late drinks and dinner, following the same "nutrition plan" you enjoyed in college. Unfortunately you're no longer twenty and spending leisurely afternoons in the gym, so your body begins to morph. The worst part of the day is stepping out of the shower and seeing the pear shape emerging in the mirror. By the time you get home from work, it's all you can do to slump in front of the TV for an hour. If you're in a relationship or trying to build one, there's no energy left for that person. You graze on more junk food before collapsing in bed for another short slumber before repeating the process the next day.

Is that you?

If not, maybe you're a stay-at-home mom, the CEO of the household. You're jolted out of bed by a screaming baby, and your first hour is a blur of dealing with an infant and perhaps getting older kids off to school. Your morning and early afternoon evaporates, a whirlwind of feedings, play dates, and diapers. By midafternoon it's time to chauffeur the kids to sports, music practice, and other extracurricular activities.

Along the way you must handle the crush of household routines, the inevitable home maintenance crisis, and the small matter of feeding yourself. By dinnertime all you've consumed is coffee and the fast-food lunch you picked up on the way back from the play date. You'd like to work off the extra pounds you've packed on in recent years, but who has the time?

Is that you?

If not, perhaps you're a woman balancing a business or corporate job with being a wife and mother. You're torn in every direction. On one hand, you perhaps feel guilt for leaving your children in the hands of your husband, a nanny, parent, or daycare service to pursue a career and provide for your family. Or perhaps you feel resentment from colleagues when you have to take time off to deal with a sick or injured child. You're supporting team members at work and a family at home, and even when you're managing to pull it off, you feel run-down, getting by on caffeine, adrenaline, and force of will.

Spartan woman? Let's see Queen Gorgo tackle this!

Even if you're a young teenage woman, with seemingly fewer responsibilities, you're feeling the pressure. Programmed for achievement at a young age, your days are overscheduled with school, extracurricular activities, and, hopefully, a social life. You wake up too late to have a substantial breakfast, if any, and because you're not allowed to eat in class, you're famished most of the morning. Had you grown up in ancient Greece, you might have been exposed to regular physical activity, but your school district cut physical education years ago. Other budget issues have forced the school to serve nothing but processed, high-starch meals and sell its soul to soda and snack companies, whose machines are everywhere.

When you finally get home, you're so hungry that you grab the first thing available, which usually is junk food. Homework, phone calls, friends, and e-mail take up the afternoon and much of the evening, which includes pizza or a takeout dinner that your parents brought home.

It's all for the greater good, or so it seems. You've probably heard of the concept of "taking one for the team" or "sacrificing your body." In baseball or softball it's when batters allow themselves to be hit by a pitch in order to get on base and perhaps start a rally. In basketball it's when a player draws a charge, allowing an opponent to essentially run over her in order to regain possession of the ball. Taking one for the team is a selfless act. You sacrifice your body for the greater goal of helping your team win.

I see women taking one for the team every day. But instead of enduring a few seconds of pain in an athletic endeavor, they're sacrificing their short-term performance and long-term health. It seems like a noble gesture. At the very least, the woman is giving up her body in pursuit of academic or career goals. She might also have a team at work counting on her or a team at home consisting of a significant other and/or children.

It's easy to rationalize ignoring proper nutrition, movement, and rest. *I can't take time for myself. There are people counting on me!*

When we talk about sacrificing the body, it's not just about losing that girlish bikini physique, though that fear is the inspiration behind most diet-and-exercise programs. There's nothing wrong with wanting to regain a lean, powerful, sexy body that's resistant to injury and long-term deterioration—or create one for the first time. This program will help you do just that.

External motivation, however, tends to be short-lived. The more powerful motivation comes from within. Not only do you want to avoid the many physical problems related to poor diet and inactivity—the short list includes diabetes, cancer, arthritis, and tendinitis—but you want to have the energy and strength to be that bedrock for your team, whatever it may be. Even if you're a single person, you don't want to short-change your performance and sabotage your personal and professional future.

One of the greatest dilemmas I hear about from women is that they feel guilty for taking time for themselves because they're so accustomed to putting the needs of others first. Again, that's an admirable position. But you cannot be successful unless you take care of yourself first. You can pull it off for a while, but this pattern of deficit spending with your health will catch up eventually. The combination of poor eating, stress, and feeling overwhelmed drives your emotional states, which changes how you fuel your body and the decisions you make regarding why you're eating and what you're eating. That, in turn, will impact your energy level, mood, and ultimately your health. It's a vicious downward spiral—with no bailout plan.

In order to help others, you must put yourself first. Think of the advice you hear from the flight attendant at the start of every flight: "If you're seated next to a child, attach your own oxygen mask first." The reasoning is that if you try to help the child first, you might run out of oxygen before you can even help the kid, let alone yourself. Those emergency instructions, which you've heard a hundred times if you fly regularly, are a terrific metaphor for life. If you don't invest in yourself first, you ultimately will not be able to support yourself or your teams. There is no way to help another person unless you first help yourself.

It's time to get back to the Core Fundamentals, to lead a Spartan existence of sorts. I've been blessed to work with some of the top female athletes in sports, as well as high-achieving women of all ages from all walks of life. The one thing they were lacking before they came to us was a support system to provide them with the same highly focused effort that they provide their own teams.

This book is your support team. Let's rediscover that Spartan woman within you together.

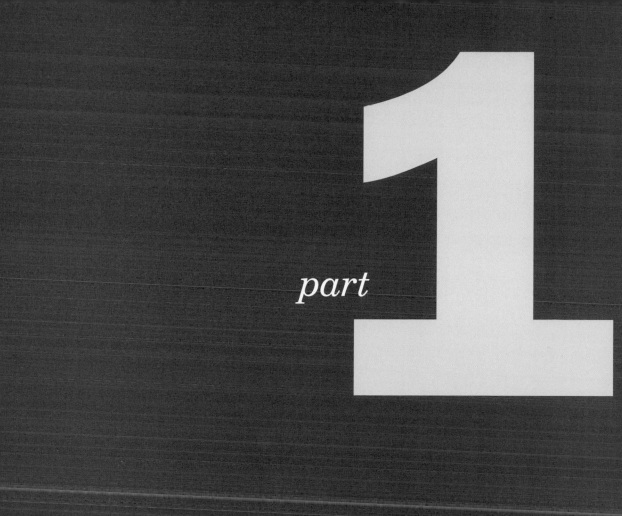

part

1

THE CORE PERFORMANCE MINDSET

THE CENTERED SELF

My coauthor, Pete Williams, and his wife have young children. There's perhaps no greater challenge and responsibility in life than raising kids. As a journalist, Pete is forever seeking information and, not surprisingly, he has sought advice from parents whose children have grown into well-mannered, responsible, high-achieving young adults.

One recent morning Pete was walking along the beach at the start of a triathlon, chatting with a middle-aged friend and fellow triathlete named Carol, who casually mentioned that the previous evening her daughter had been offered a full swimming scholarship to a major Division I university.

Pete noticed the number 53 written on the back of Carol's right calf, signifying her age. Like many triathletes, she looks much younger. Pete offered hearty congratulations. What a remarkable accomplishment for Carol, her husband, and, of course, their daughter. As they waded into the water to warm up for the race, Pete asked if there was one piece of advice she could offer on how she raised such a motivated self-starter of a child, let alone a Division I athlete.

Pete figured Carol and her husband had introduced the girl to swim lessons early. Perhaps they hired special coaches, sacrificed weekends and vacations to attend swim meets, and otherwise dedicated a huge chunk of their lives to swimming.

"All of that is true," Carol said. "But none of it would have mattered if my daughter had not from a young age seen me getting up early to swim and train and the positive impact it had on every aspect of my life. She's always looked at me as this Energizer Bunny and realized early on that I'm like this because of the way I eat, train, and the attitude I have."

Carol adjusted her swim goggles and waded in deeper. "If you set a good example, you won't have to push your kids," she said. "They'll get the message."

As an accomplished professional, mother, and age-group triathlon competitor, Carol is an example of a woman who recognizes that she can perform at her best and thus best serve her loved ones *by putting herself first*.

Let me explain. Women, to a fault, tend to put others first. They traditionally shoulder most of the burden of social organization, child-rearing, and household management. They provide the emotional backbone for their families and friends. As a result, they often feel overwhelmed.

Women need to focus more on being what I call a "centered self." This is the opposite of being self-centered. By focusing first on your Core Fundamentals of Mindset, Nutrition, Movement, and Recovery, you'll be in better position to serve those around you.

Financial advisors are forever preaching the notion of "paying yourself first," immediately taking a percentage of each paycheck—no matter how small—and socking it away in savings or investments, even before paying bills. Inevitably you spend less and still have enough funds to pay your expenses. Not only that, you become wealthier through the miracle of compound interest and (hopefully) a reasonable return on your investments.

On the other hand, if you first pay bills and take care of other expenses, it's funny how there's nothing left to save and invest. You're tapped out, not sure where all the cash went.

The same is true with your time, the only fixed asset we share. We each have the same twenty-four-hour day. If we wait to allocate time to adequately address our Mindset, Nutrition, Movement, and Recovery, there never will be enough hours in the day. By the time we take care of work, family and friends, and the daily chores of life, there's no time remaining.

In each of these Core Fundamental areas—Mindset, Nutrition, Movement, and Recovery—it's possible to better allocate time to create *more* time. By generating more energy and moving through life more efficiently, you'll perform better and discover more time for what's most important.

Let's use Movement as an example, since the objection I hear most is "I don't have time to get to the gym."

We need to stop looking at training our bodies as a luxury but a necessity, like saving for the future. Just as there are things you need to do to be competent at your job, there are things necessary to perform in the game of life. If I told you that a professional athlete was going to take the field but had done nothing to prepare, you would expect her to fail. So why should a young professional or parent expect to just show up and be prepared for success that day?

"Now, wait just a minute," you might say. "I'm a lawyer and I spend countless hours preparing for client meetings, depositions, and appearances in the courtroom. Nobody is better prepared than I am. Every day I know I'm going to kick some major legal butt regardless of whether I hit the gym or eat a chicken breast and a salad."

Fair enough. But will you be able to repeat this performance day after day, month after month, and year after year? Could it be you're getting by mostly on caffeine, adrenaline, and force of will? Are you positive you're performing at your best?

It could be that your performance has been declining so gradually you're not even aware of it. If you've ever owned an expensive, high-end vacuum cleaner, you're familiar with this process. These machines are terrific when they're new. They suck up everything, to the point where you're embarrassed how dirty your house was. But if you don't religiously clean the filters, they gradually lose power. You might not notice this as it's happening because you put more and more effort into vacuuming your floors, until one day the vacuum does not pick up anything.

The same is true with your body, which has an uncanny ability to compensate and pick up slack, albeit by putting undue pressure on joints from lack of proper movement and by suffering internally from poor nutrition.

Like that vacuum cleaner, your body has the potential to be an incredible high-performance machine. But if you ignore routine maintenance, let alone the opportunity to make it perform better, it will break down and require some costly, time-consuming repairs.

Most people who own high-end vacuum cleaners spend a small amount of time after each use on cleaning filters and other routine maintenance. Many people are downright obsessive-compulsive about taking care of their automobiles, adhering to all manner of 3,000-, 10,000-, and 30,000-mile maintenance programs. Yet they run their bodies hard, like rental cars they can turn in at the end of the week, assuming they'll operate well forever.

It's one thing to run a car or vacuum cleaner into the ground; they're replaceable. You only have one body, one "vehicle for success," and though it's possible to replace certain original parts (hip, knee, etc.), it's expensive, painful, and undesirable.

By building a strong foundation of Mindset, Nutrition, Movement, and Recovery, you'll have the energy necessary to succeed and the ability to prevent this downward spiral. If you don't establish this foundation, you might be able to get by for a period of time without investing back in yourself, but you will be deficit spending with your health.

What do I mean by deficit spending? It's the process of compromising your long-term health for short-term energy. It's no different than tapping into reserve funds for today's living expenses. Just as investors want to build for the future while meeting the demands of today, we want to create the energy we need to thrive in the moment while investing in our long-term health and success.

Here's how deficit spending works. If you eat poorly, feel stressed and over-whelmed, and struggle to take time for yourself, it's going to affect your emotional state. That, in turn, impacts how you fuel your body and the decisions you make regarding why you're eating and what you're eating. The stress and diet contribute to an inability to rest and decreased quality of sleep, which create more stress.

This program is not going to produce a stress-free life. I'm not sure that would be desirable, even if it were an option. What this program *will* do is give you a sound foundation so that when life gets stressful, you can pull back and focus on those Core Fundamental practices of Mindset, Nutrition, Movement, and Recovery.

This really isn't any different from other aspects of your life for which I'm sure you do a tremendous job of planning, whether it's financial or retirement planning, saving for college, or simply getting ready for a vacation.

In all of those areas, you can see steady progress. It's easy to quantify in financial statements or how much everyone enjoyed the vacation. The professional athletes I work with need look only at a scoreboard and hear the roar of the crowd for immediate feedback.

How well are you doing with your Mindset, Nutrition, Movement, and Recovery? It's not as simple as getting a clean bill of health from the doctor or the reading on the scale. Those can be helpful indicators, but then again it's also possible to run a car for many thousands of miles without doing any preventive maintenance. Unless you're investing in yourself, as you would with regular auto maintenance, you don't know for sure how you're doing.

Your life is much tougher than that of a pro athlete because there is no massive support team handling everything for you and no feedback system. If you're a mother, you've made a 24/7 commitment for a minimum of eighteen years. There are no screaming fans to motivate you. Screaming children, yes, but no coach to guide you, no annual job evaluation or performance review.

The sad part is that you perform this valuable but often thankless job of child-rearing for eighteen years and you still don't know for sure what kind of job you did until perhaps another eighteen years pass and you look up one day and say, "Hey, my kids turned out to be good people; I did a pretty good job."

It's a massive challenge, regardless of where you are in life. This program is your support team, your strategy to tackle the "game of life," whether you're a single person or someone responsible for a significant other and/or kids. Either way, it takes a tremendous amount of focus, energy, and organization. If that game plan doesn't include supporting you, it's going to be very difficult to reach those goals.

Remember that discussion from the previous chapter about "sacrificing your body"? This isn't just about putting on the "freshman fifteen" at college, struggling to lose baby weight, or dealing with a middle-age spread. All of those are legitimate concerns. The real sacrifice can be seen in elderly women who have been so diligent in serving children and grandchildren that their bodies are ruined. They're exhausted and suffering from obesity, which leads to diabetes and other significant ailments, even cancer. They're prone to osteoporosis and every "itis" imaginable, including arthritis, tendinitis, and bursitis.

These women have worked their entire lives to reach what should be the golden years. They're empty nesters, financially secure, and in a place where they should be able to enjoy a high quality of life. Instead they're paying the price with aches and pains that don't allow them to enjoy the retirement they envisioned thirty years earlier. They spend their days traipsing from one doctor's office to another and much of their fixed incomes are spent on medications.

This would be unacceptable to me were it just the elderly. But it's also happening to women at younger and younger ages all the time. It wasn't that long ago when if you saw someone confined to a wheelchair, it was because that person was a war veteran or injured in an automobile accident. These days many people need wheelchairs as a result of conditions brought on by a lifetime of poor eating and a lack of movement.

Much of this is preventable, and it's not too late—or early—to start. We want to reverse the clock and implement these strategies that we know will enable women to enjoy a high quality of life well into their senior years. An improvement in Mindset, Nutrition, Movement, and Recovery truly can be a Fountain of Youth.

Let's get back to Pete's friend Carol, the triathlete and swimming mom. She invests time several mornings a week to train. She follows a high-performance nutrition program that, along with her training and proper mindset, fuels her body for greater success. Not only does she look ten years younger, she has none of the injuries and nagging ailments common to women her age. She takes no medications.

Carol is more efficient and productive at work, getting more accomplished than her colleagues in less time. She rarely needs to stay late, and when she arrives home she is less beaten down by the stress of the day than her coworkers are. As a result, she has more energy left to share with her husband and two daughters. That small investment she makes in nutrition and training pays off tenfold.

Best of all, Carol serves as a glowing example to her children, who, like their mom, are high achievers. Unlike many of their classmates, they understand the necessity of following a proper nutrition program, getting enough sleep and other recovery, and training their bodies to thrive in the game of life.

Their friends marvel at how much the girls accomplish even though they have active social lives. Yet Carol's daughters don't drink coffee or energy drinks, or rely on

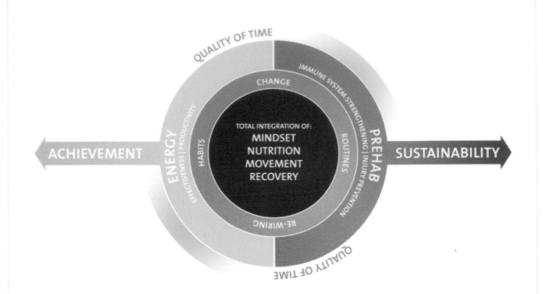

This diagram was developed in collaboration with our partners at Tignum, the world's leading institute for sustainable performance.

vending machines to get through the day. They have healthy skin, lean, fit bodies, and the energy to tackle any challenge.

The formula, which the girls are happy to share with friends, is quite simple. By following this system of Mindset, Nutrition, Movement, and Recovery, they are able to get more done in less time and do it more efficiently.

These are the Core Fundamentals of the Core Performance system, the "core of the core," if you will. The Core Performance system is not to be confused with abdominal routines or quick-fix training solutions popularized by the mainstream media, forever in search of a simple, digestible sound bite.

Instead, let's think of your core as a Super Ball, the small red rubber ball that you might find if you cut open a baseball. As a kid I used to love getting Super Balls out of the gumball machine (I know I'm dating myself here) and slamming them against the ground. I marveled at the power of the Super Ball as it soared seemingly ten stories in the air, hit the ground, and rose once again.

We want to create a Super Ball in your own core, not just through nutrition and training but by rewiring your mindset and incorporating recovery into your lifestyle. Let's take a brief look at each of these four components.

MINDSET: Most diet-and-exercise programs assume that if you eat right and get into better shape, everything else will take care of itself. Aside from a lucky and dedicated few, that only works for the short term; most of us need a game plan to keep us going. After all, even the most physically gifted athletes cannot succeed unless they have mentally addressed everything they will face in competition. Developing the proper mindset will help prepare you for everything that comes your way. To do this, it's necessary to examine what motivates you. What are the roles you play in life and what's most important? Who is relying upon you? What are the long-term goals that will keep you committed to this sustainable Core Performance program? We'll answer those questions in the next chapter.

NUTRITION: If you're hoping for an exotic signature diet to emerge from these pages, you're going to be disappointed. What I can tell you is that you're going to discover a simple, sustainable nutrition plan for the rest of your life, one that will leave you energized and fueled for high performance.

We're going to change your approach to eating. Instead of living to eat, we're going to eat to live. Instead of using food to change your emotional state or deal with stress, you're going to use it to fuel your body for maximum performance. It's not just about looking good in that swimsuit, which you'll also accomplish by the way.

Instead you're going to use food to fuel your success and sustain your energy level. Not only that, but by planning to eat properly and putting a game plan in place, you'll also save time and money.

MOVEMENT: I'm not a fan of the word *exercise*. It's come to refer to slow, repetitive, nonchallenging activity. You might take your pooch to the "Dog Exercise

Area," though our canine friends tend to exert themselves far more than humans who exercise.

I prefer the term *movement*, since it's more indicative of an active lifestyle. Not only that, it's indicative of the proper way to move your body. I know plenty of people who "exercise" with poor movement patterns that inevitably lead to injury and long-term ailments. That's what we want to avoid. In this program you'll train your body for proper movement, in effect becoming a powerful Super Ball.

RECOVERY: American culture fosters a mindset of working longer and longer, the idea being that the more we work, the more we accomplish. That's not really the case. We want to work more efficiently, getting more done in less time.

I cringe whenever I hear someone say, "I give 110 percent every day." That's impossible. Just as we need proper sleep every day, we need to work recovery into every week, month, and year.

After all, it's impossible to maintain the pace of twelve-hour days without your body breaking down. Throughout this program you'll learn the importance of recovery, or what I like to call *regeneration*.

Regeneration applies to everything: Mindset, Nutrition, and Movement. You can't work out hard six days a week: Your body will break down. So we've constructed this program with hard days and easier "regeneration days" that allow you time to recover.

The same is true with nutrition. If I gave you an all-or-nothing diet of healthy foods, you would quickly fall off the wagon. So there will be recovery periods that allow you to indulge in foods that might not be especially healthy but that you really enjoy.

Regeneration also applies to your mindset. The primary purpose of a vacation is for your mind to recover from the grind of everyday life. We need to build these breaks into our lives in order to come back even stronger.

These four components—Mindset, Nutrition, Movement, and Recovery—do not operate independently. Core Performance for Women is an integrated program that will serve as the framework for every aspect of your life. Let's begin with establishing that proper mindset.

CHAPTER 1 SUMMARY: Successful women recognize that in order to perform well, it's necessary to place themselves first. By taking care of the Core Fundamentals of Mindset, Nutrition, Movement, and Recovery, you'll be more efficient and productive in all aspects of your lives and be able to create more time and energy to support loved ones. By working all four pillars of the Core Performance system, you can produce the energy and structure to thrive.

ROLE PLAYING

Consider for a moment your current stage of life. Regardless of where you are, think of yourself as a powerful force for producing change in the lives of others. Now ask yourself what you do each day to build those powers. Not just in your career, but in terms of making yourself into the person you want to be. What are the core values that drive you?

If you turned to this chapter expecting to delve into the Nutrition and Movement portion of the program, perhaps this exercise might seem unnecessary, even a little touchy-feely. After all, we live in a quick-fix world, where it's easy to say, "Tell me what to do and let's get on with it. I'm here, I'm motivated and ready to work."

That's a great attitude to have. At the same time, it stops short of creating the proper mindset for success. That's because people approach traditional diet-and-exercise programs much like remodeling a house. They want the transformation to be as quick and dramatic as possible. The emphasis is more on the transformation rather than on implementing a sustainable solution.

I love watching home improvement shows on HGTV. It's amazing what motivated homeowners, working with skilled designers and carpenters, can create in a short period of time. But as a fairly handy guy who has done some remodeling myself, I sometimes shake my head at the results. The craftsmanship is usually top-notch, but the design and color schemes are often too trendy, something that will look out-of-date in a few years. The materials are high maintenance or not meant to last more than a couple of years. I often wonder if the homeowner is satisfied with the results three years later.

The homeowner was motivated by producing an eye-popping, dramatic change, perhaps at the expense of a more timeless, low-maintenance, longer-lasting design. There's nothing wrong with a dramatic renovation. But sometimes it tends to be a checklist item, like getting in the best shape of your life for a wedding, reunion, or vacation. That motivation tends to be external and short-lived.

Among the many reasons why most nutrition-and-exercise programs do not produce lasting change is that people view their health as something to be renovated, a remodeling project with a definitive beginning and end. They want the fastest, easiest possible solution and, failing that, there's always plastic surgery and liposuction.

People tend to make changes from the outside in. But unless you make fundamental alterations, overhauling your mindset, it's just short-term, until one day you wake up not quite sure who you are, where you've been, or where you want to go.

In the last chapter we talked about creating this *centered self,* building from the inside and moving out. Many women (and men) take the opposite approach, committing to quick starvation diets that might take off weight but damage their insides through nutrient deprivation. Instead of losing fat, they lose positive lean mass, which burns more calories and is the engine of a healthy physique. These women are what I call "skinny fat," thin but with high levels of body fat and lacking in the type of energy-sustaining lean mass that truly looks good in a swimsuit.

Other people fall prey to the dangers of "body acceptance." Now I will be the first to say that it is a terrible thing when people are ostracized or discriminated against for being overweight. I understand the notion of being comfortable in one's own skin, no matter how much of it there is, and there's no question that the notion of the BBW (big beautiful woman) is here to stay. Many overweight women and men remain over-weight because they know their partners will love them regardless of their size.

At the same time, acceptance of one's own body can lead to long-term ailments and disease, to say nothing of affecting quality of life and performance. Accepting others for who they are is an important core value, but it doesn't mean you have to accept your current body as a life sentence. In fact, it could be a death sentence. If you're enduring this extra weight, chances are you're not able to perform your best, let alone serve your loved ones as best you could. Why not provide them with a better you?

If you're someone in this position, you've probably forgotten what it's like to be firing on all cylinders, to have boundless energy, and to be operating with optimal power. You've adjusted to life at half speed rather than living and thriving at full throttle.

Once you can make the connection between how you fuel and train your body and what you're able to accomplish with this greater energy, that's a powerful thing. It becomes a life force when you recognize how this energy enables you to live your dreams and better serve others, especially the ones you hold most dear.

Regardless of where you are in life, you have the potential to be a driving force in your life and the lives of others. As a woman, you will play at least one of the following roles throughout your life:

SELF

PROFESSIONAL

SPOUSE/PARTNER (MOTHER)

Some women take on all of these roles over the course of their lives, sometimes all at once. Others move between the roles. Regardless of where you are along the road of life, you're always going to have the role of self.

The self stage is where we define our core values and what we want out of life. Here we map out our vision and create our definition of success. Early on it's an individualized, self-centered vision as you move through high school, perhaps college, and young adulthood.

Even if there's no significant other or family at this stage, you still have your role as self and are part of a professional family of sorts. Here, too, you must have these same core values and core fundamentals to fuel your success. Beyond the self and young professional stage there's the other possible variable of family and friends, where the energy and effort you put into those relationships is going to be another one of your roles.

Regardless of who you are, you will play the role of self. You may choose to have this working side of life, whether it's working for someone else or being the head of your own business. The third role could be having a significant other and having a family. Here you'll likely add the title of CEO of the household, either on a full-time basis or sharing it with a significant other, or juggling it with a career outside the home.

We live in a fast-paced, hectic world where it's challenging enough just to master the self role, let alone add the roles of professional, spouse/significant other, and perhaps mother. Futurists predict that there might be thirty or forty paradigm shifts in the next fifty years requiring massive adjustments by everyone. By comparison, there have been only two or three paradigm shifts over the last five decades. All we know is that change will be constant, and we need to have a deeper understanding and stability of self.

When we begin to add professional responsibilities to the self role, recognizing the rapid pace of business and the adaptations it requires, it creates a massive challenge. By adding some combination of friends, a significant other, and family to the mix, you're now wearing three major hats, and that takes tremendous focus.

I work with professional athletes and am reminded daily of the commitment and sacrifice they must make to perform at their best. At least they have a massive support system in place. Our goal with this program is to give you a support mechanism for success, first for yourself, then as a professional, and ultimately so that you can make the others around you more successful.

This is a lifelong evolution. When you're young it's all about trying to please other people. Kids keep their rooms clean and get good grades to make Mom happy. Teenagers and young women exercise and eat right to fit into smaller jeans and attract a mate. This "outside-in" approach helps you reach your goals of being accepted and fitting in or finding the fulfilling things in life.

The switch to an "inside-out" approach has to come, and the sooner the better. The idea is to discover the beauty and energy within and let it express itself externally. That's what the Core Performance for Women system is all about. It's not about being self-centered and doing whatever it takes to impress or attract others. Instead, it's about being a centered self and building this success from the inside out on the cellular level, from brain to body. That's where we want to be.

For some people, the internal motivation does not come until they've brought a significant other or even children into the equation. When they're living a single lifestyle of partying that could lead to obesity, diabetes, eating disorders, and other ailments, it's easier to rationalize. After all, they're only hurting themselves. But once you have others depending on you, it's a lot more motivating. You can either elevate others or pull those people into the same downward spiral. Most people in this situation feel a sense of responsibility to be there for those people. Sometimes the trigger is a teary-eyed child begging a parent to stop smoking, drinking, or eating destructively because they want them to be around.

Wanting to be around to watch your children grow up and see grandchildren is the ultimate motivation for some people. Grandparents often have the time and resources to provide things they never could as parents, and that can be a wonderful gift. But you probably won't want to be around if you can't get out of a chair or struggle with pain so much that you'll be a burden to your offspring.

This program always comes back to Mindset and understanding your definition of success. That's what will provide lasting motivation, not fitting into smaller jeans or a swimsuit. Even if you've never defined success, I'm guessing deep down that you know what your vision of real accomplishment is and what you want to create. We all have core values that we do not want to compromise. Every day we're faced with choices, and it takes strength and courage to make the right decisions as you make your way toward your best self.

When I work with professional athletes, their goals are a little easier to define. They want to play as long as possible, perform beyond their wildest dreams, and win championships. Their sport has a defined set of movement patterns, perhaps even more specialized if they play a certain position within that game.

I don't know what specific roles you play, the goals you have, or your definition of success. But I do know your roles fall into the three categories discussed above. I imagine you're looking for a sustainable program to provide greater energy and a lean physique that's resistant to injury and long-term deterioration. Who doesn't want that?

Together we can develop the greatest game plan in the world, but if it does not resonate with you emotionally and mentally based on this definition of success, we're unlikely to succeed.

What is that definition of success? Is it watching a child get married or playing

The Meaning of Success

What is your definition of success?

What roles do you play at home, at work?

What drives you?

What would the people you touch through your various roles say about you today, as opposed to what you'd like them to say about you in a eulogy?

What changes do you need to create so that they would say what you would like to hear in your eulogy?

with grandkids? Is it a certain level of professional and financial accomplishment? Does it include community involvement, travel, or hobbies? Once we're able to define it and commit to it, then we can go side by side in this journey. If it's a matter of me telling you what this journey is going to be, that's not going to produce long-term results. That's outside-in motivation. Instead, let's focus on building this "vehicle for success" from the inside out.

Through "The Meaning of Success" and "What Roles Do You Play?" exercises described here, you are going to commit to change your mindset, which will give you tangible goals based on the best possible you, not on how you look or how much you make. Take a moment now and create your own meaning of success through these exercises. Instead of writing in the book, use a separate sheet of paper and keep it in a place where you can review it regularly. Our Core Performance "KISS" principle is to keep it short and simple; this is an instance where less often is more.

Your definition of success is going to change as you progress through this journey of life. It evolves from high school to college and further as you navigate the professional world, which is often the first experience with taking on serious responsibility. There might be additional responsibilities with a significant other or perhaps as a mother.

It doesn't matter what your definition of success is. What's important is that it

What Roles Do You Play?

What are your roles?

What do you need to do for each of these roles? What is the definition of success needed to improve the quality of each one of these roles in life?

Ask yourself: What will make you feel successful in the areas of mental, physical, and spiritual development?

What will make you feel successful in the important role you play for your spouse or significant other?

What do you need to be successful in your role with your family—as a daughter, sister, or mother?

What role do you fill with your friends? How can you fill this role more successfully?

What is your role with your colleagues at work, at school, in the organizations you're involved with?

will point the way to fulfillment. The only thing we can be assured of is that life will knock us down, and we need to have the resilience to get back up or get back on the right path to fulfill that definition of success for that point in time.

As you do the exercise above, ask yourself what you need to fulfill each of the roles you play. What role do you play for your spouse or significant other? What roles do you play to make the relationship special? Once you've defined your roles, ask yourself what other people would say about you in these roles. Would your spouse say that you don't make enough time, or that you are not engaged enough when you do? What would you want your spouse or significant other to say?

What would your friends say about you? Would they say that you're there for them when they need you? Or would they say that they're tired of hearing about all of your problems, about how life has been unfair? How about your coworkers? Would they say you're a nice person? Would they think you're productive and effective at work or someone who drags down the office?

If you work in an office or go to school, would your colleagues say that you goof off too much? Or have you found the happy medium and are able to buckle down when you have to but don't take yourself too seriously? Are you known for laughing and having fun or for being stressed out and holding on too tight?

In short, what do you want people to think or say about you? Go back to each of the roles listed above. Are you setting a good example? Are you comfortable with the way you're perceived?

What does all of this have to do with Nutrition and Movement? In a word: everything. Going through these exercises gives you a sense of your true north and gives you added motivation to move toward a long-term success plan. But, more important, you'll come to recognize that this isn't just about you—you're undertaking this transformation to better serve and elevate the people you care about most. This takes a lot of energy, which can only be generated by committing to this program.

Once we've defined success and considered the roles we play, it's easier to start looking at ourselves from the perspective of the centered self rather than being self-centered. By embarking on this process, you're going to be better able to lift your friends and family, but it starts with you.

Now that we've laid the groundwork for our Mindset, let's start by properly fueling your body, the vehicle for your success. In the next section, we'll start with the Core Nutrition program—everything you need to know to develop and maintain a high-performance diet.

Though Nutrition comes before Movement, I don't mean to imply that one is more important than the other. I'm always discouraged when people embark on diets without implementing any sort of Movement patterns into their lives. I understand why it happens. After all, everyone has to eat, but exercise is optional (though it shouldn't

CORE WOMEN SUCCESS STORY

"Tall in the Saddle."

Sue Ross • Age: Fifty • Hometown: Topanga, California

As Sue Ross approached the age of fifty, she noticed that her body no longer rebounded from intense activity the way it did years earlier. Whether working in the yard, training in the gym, or engaging her passion of equestrian dressage events, she would feel pain in her lower back and right knee as well as soreness all over.

Core strength is especially important in dressage, where horse and rider move as one unit and are judged by their ability to execute a formal sequence of movements. For the rider it's essential to have a strong core and perfect posture so she can feel relaxed but still influence the horse by subtle weight movements.

A 120-pound rider like Ross is no match for a 1,200-pound horse, but she says having improved core strength has helped her stay at the top of her game—and on top of the horse.

"Core strength is so important because you need to be able to sit down into the horse and not let him pull you," says Ross, a human resources director. "At the same time, you must not pull on him either."

Ross never thought of herself as an athlete, just a middle-aged woman with a busy schedule trying to avoid adding extra pounds. Just listening to a friend's tales of running and ocean swimming left her exhausted.

Though Ross worked out regularly at a local gym, she never felt the energy and core strength that her friend seemed to have. That was before her friend introduced her to the Core Performance program via the Core Performance Center in Santa Monica, California.

Ross embraced the program's integrated,

holistic approach of Mindset, Nutrition, Movement, and Recovery and was stunned to feel changes in flexibility, strength, and mobility immediately. After twelve training sessions, the changes were dramatic.

"I made great strides in terms of my core strength, posture, hip flexibility, and balance," she says. "It was a fantastic sense of achievement to see the measurable progress I had made in a relatively short period of time."

Even though she competed in a sport that placed a premium on perfectly executed movements, Ross never considered the connection between improper movement and physical pain.

"I thought the aches and pains I felt after working out or that were part of my daily life were a product of getting older and wear and tear on the body," she says. "The Core Performance program has strengthened my body and taught me how to use it more correctly. I rarely feel my right knee anymore, when before it would cause me a great deal of discomfort after a workout; it had never occurred to me that I might not be using it correctly or that compensating for other parts of my body could cause this type of soreness."

Perhaps the most telling result of her new training regimen came one afternoon when she installed more than one hundred plants in her yard. Before she adopted the Core Performance regimen, such bending and reaching would have resulted in a sore lower back.

"It occurred to me that I had not experienced any discomfort," Ross said. "The training has strengthened my lower back and taught me how to move properly to the extent that I can now enjoy simple functional movements that previously would have given me problems.

"I'm still not sure if I'll ever call myself an athlete, but I know I'll continue to benefit from the Core workouts both in my equestrian activities and everyday life."

be). You get so much more out of the nutrition program when you exercise—and vice versa.

I've made the workout program in this book as effective and time-efficient as possible. I understand the hectic lives of women of all ages. If there are times when you can't follow the training regimen, then at least stick to the nutrition portion. That alone will improve your health significantly.

It would be tempting to title this book "The Core Diet" or "The Core Diet for Women." That seems to be what the marketing folks prefer and no doubt would attract the folks who wander from one fad diet to another, seeking remodeling tips rather than a strong foundation. But even though we're intensely proud of the research we've done in the field of nutrition, that would be shortchanging the rest of the program and grouping *Core Performance Women* with all of those short-term fad diets that are unsustainable.

As you'll see in the next chapters, the power of Core Nutrition is that it's not a diet at all.

CHAPTER 2 SUMMARY: Successful women are guided by core values that propel them toward long-term success. By investing in ourselves first and becoming centered selves, seeking to serve family members and friends, it's possible to create powerful, sustainable motivation. Establishing a proper mindset involves defining success and recognizing the roles you play which, in turn, help keep you on track with training and nutrition.

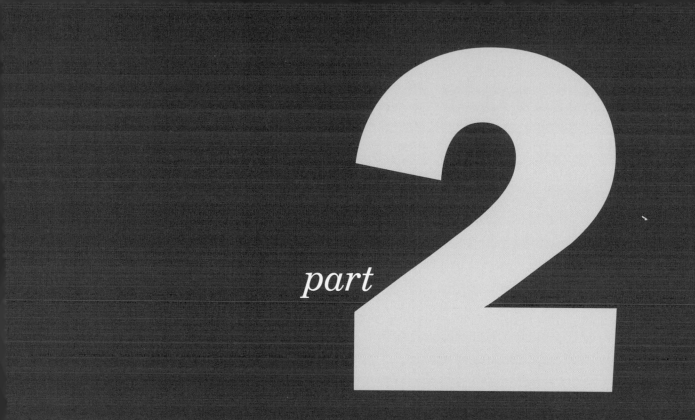

## part 2

CORE PERFORMANCE WOMEN NUTRITION

THE ENERGY CRISIS

I sometimes marvel at the paradigm shifts that have occurred just in my lifetime, some good, some not so good. As a child of the 1970s and early 1980s, I lived in a world where caffeine played a much, much smaller role than it does today.

Back then it seemed like nobody under the age of forty drank coffee. Television commercials for Folgers, Maxwell House, and Taster's Choice featured middle-aged folks and seniors debating the merits of various blends. Though Starbucks was founded in 1971, its owners initially intended their business to be selling beans for home brewing. It was another twenty years before Starbucks began to grow into the colossus it is today, offering coffee on the go from every street corner.

Back in my youth Coca-Cola and Pepsi already were big companies, but soda for most people was a treat, not an everyday beverage. Heck, Diet Coke was not introduced until 1982.

As for so-called energy drinks, there were so few they weren't considered a category. As recently as twenty years ago the few that existed, like Jolt cola, were used mostly by college students pulling all-nighters. Now we have Red Bull and dozens of similar heavily caffeinated beverages—in sugar-laden and nonsugar varieties—that are consumed routinely by people of all ages, all day, every day. Everyone, including teenagers, is pounding energy drinks and coffee.

How did we suddenly run out of energy, especially when we know so much more about nutrition now than we did in the days of disco?

Back then moms talked about how "breakfast is the most important meal of the day," which is still true. During school health classes kids learned about the importance of "three square meals" and "the four food groups." Those philosophies have been updated since, but at least back then kids were getting some sort of nutrition education.

Most families gathered around the dinner table each evening. Eating out for most was not an everyday occurrence. There were no fern bar restaurants, few "fast casual" dining establishments, and even pizza delivery was far from the multibillion dollar business it is today.

This wasn't that long ago, just the mid-1980s. But things changed quickly. As more women entered the workforce, the traditional family dinner disappeared. Grabbing takeout and eating out became commonplace. Eating on the go or while doing something else—watching television, working, even driving—became the norm. Parents and kids no longer left home in the morning with a bag lunch, opting instead to buy a midday meal that usually offered less nutritional value, though more calories.

Along the way nutrition education suffered. Kids grew up learning from their parents that eating out or consuming packaged processed foods was the norm. As schools began to eliminate physical education classes, they also cut health instruction, introduced vending machines, and partnered with fast-food chains to diversify the school food offerings, further eroding the nutritional knowledge base. The influence of the mass media and food marketers on our food choices grew exponentially.

Meanwhile, our food became more processed, and our beef, poultry, and dairy products were injected with growth hormones and fed a diet of corn. Artificial sweeteners like high-fructose corn syrup (HFCS) began popping up in everything we commonly consume, from cookies and crackers to bread and ketchup. No longer did people prepare their own food. After all, why take the time to make something yourself when someone else could make it for you?

This paradigm shift in nutrition coincided with an even bigger one in technology that took kids out of the backyard and playground and placed them in front of video games, cable television, and computers. Instead of spending their afternoons actively engaged outside, they sat indoors in front of screens, often with snack foods.

Parents, meanwhile, discovered that the nine-to-five workday was no more. They worked longer hours, eating when and what they could, and spending less time moving their bodies. Evenings, once considered family or hobby time, became focused on television and, later, the Internet.

Everyone, it seemed, was working longer, sleeping less, and eating far differently than people did in the 1970s.

The solution? Takeout food and caffeine. Lots of caffeine.

Don't get me wrong; there's a place for coffee and caffeine. I'm a big fan of the customer service provided by Starbucks and I wish more industries made such a commitment. The problem is that you have people trying to do more in less time, with fuel devoid of nutrients. They're mindlessly reaching for energy in the form of caffeine and sugar, whether they're getting it from coffee, empty calories, or from energy drinks, which are loaded with massive doses of caffeine and neural stimulants. In many respects they're no different than nicotine—drugs that provide short-term stimulation.

I'd like to see this book offered for sale alongside energy drinks, because that's what we're providing: energy. People are buying energy drinks and spending tons of money at Starbucks because they're exhausted, and not just because of professional and personal demands. Most people don't get adequate nutrients in their diet. They're not well hydrated and they don't get quality sleep, simply because of what they consume. They don't have a nutrition plan, let alone a lifestyle program, in place to sustain optimum performance.

When you load up on caffeine, you stimulate the brain, which tells the adrenal glands to produce more adrenaline so you have more energy. So your body keeps chugging along, at least until you feed it more caffeine. Some people use so much caffeine that they experience anxiety in the evening and consume alcohol to take the edge off. If you were to treat your car this way, feeding it gas but not oil and other lubricants, it eventually would break down.

So, too, will your body. By relying on caffeine your brain becomes convinced that that's all it needs and it creates a vicious downward spiral. So many people begin their days by confusing coffee with food. Their "breakfasts" consist solely of coffee and perhaps something high in sugar, like a Danish, scone, or even a bowl of their favorite cereal. They can't function without the caffeine and sugar. Their sleep quality is poor because they don't have the proper mix of nutrients in their diet. Then the destructive cycle continues as they continue to eat poorly because they are exhausted from not getting enough quality sleep and nutrients. This is before we even start to think about how stress, travel, and relationships affect the way we eat and our energy status.

It's difficult for the brain to operate without proper nutrients. Without them you're not going to be productive for extended periods. There are studies that suggest that many people are only effective at work for four hours out of every eight-hour (or ten-hour) day.

Developing that muscle of focus and concentration takes practice; you also need the right combination of nutrients to flow through your body so you can concentrate.

Attention-Deficit Hyperactivity Disorder (ADHD) is a condition supported by science. But there are many people who diagnose themselves with ADHD because they have inconsistent energy levels as a result of poor nutrient intake and excessive sugar and/or caffeine.

I marvel how many kids today turn to energy drinks and Starbucks beverages. They should *not* be having issues with energy. If you're over the age of thirty-five, think back to when you were a kid. Did you have a problem with not having enough energy? Obviously you went through a lethargic period in your teenage years when you were going through hormonal changes, but other than that energy probably was not an issue.

Again, there's nothing wrong with caffeine. It's a powerful stimulant to have in your arsenal. But you shouldn't be relying on caffeine just to get through your day. Use it as an emergency fund to tap into in the event your child kept you up all night or you didn't travel well on a business trip. Or you could use caffeine before a big workout, knowing that you're going to expend more energy. Then it becomes an ergogenic aid, not life support. When you minimize your caffeine intake, caffeine then becomes a powerful energy boost for the times when you really need it.

I use caffeine as an example because it's indicative of the destructive nutritional patterns people fall into that ultimately rob them of energy and optimum performance. It's hardly the only such behavior. Relying on processed foods high in sugar, calories, and fat but void of nutrients to get you through the day is just as dangerous, if not more so.

It's important to recognize that the way you fuel your body is going to have an impact on your entire day. The nutrients you decide to eat and the delivery form that you choose them in will directly affect the way you think, feel, and act. That quick bowl of sugary cereal might seem like an effective way to start the morning. But it will spike your sugar and insulin levels, to the point where your body is going to crash within ninety minutes. Your focus and attention will be lower, your mood worse. That's going to affect how you act in class or at work, how you process and retain information, and how you perform. That bowl of sugary cereal will sabotage your next meal, since you will crave more sugar, resulting in a greater caloric intake over the course of the day.

There's also the issue of the quality of lunch you're eating. People tend to understand what's good nutritionally and what isn't, that vegetables and whole foods are better than processed sugars, but they don't often think about it in terms of how it's going to impact their performance. Whether you are grabbing whatever is closest because you are starving and out of time, taking something prepackaged from home, or opting for something to purchase at school or work, you risk your meal not being everything it needs to be to get you through the rest of your afternoon.

This extends to after-school and after-work activities as well. If you're training after work or picking kids up from school and taking them to music or sports practice, have you provided them and yourself with proper fuel? At this point blood sugar is probably way down, after all, and nobody is going to perform well without some fuel. Did you plan a nutritious snack or are you going to stop at a convenience store or coffee shop for a quick jolt of caffeine or sugar? When I was growing up, kids never drank coffee beverages and consumed soda only on certain occasions, perhaps following an athletic competition.

Thankfully, we know now that soda is a poor choice for post-workout consumption, but at least back then kids weren't relying on caffeine just to get through the day. The reason why many kids are relying so much on caffeine is because they're mimicking their parents, who have lost sight of what constitutes proper nutrition, which produces sufficient energy to get you through the day without caffeine. It's not that they're missing calories; the calories are missing the vital nutrients they need to support a developing body. The kids are tired and undernourished—not underfed.

We're sending our kids—and often ourselves—into the "game of life" without proper fuel. Parents insist that kids work hard in school and prepare thoroughly at home, but do we ensure that they've fueled their bodies properly for success? I'm amazed at how many parents spend big money on top-notch athletic gear but send their kids into practice or games either on empty stomachs or fueled by fast food or processed junk.

Where are people getting their information about nutrition? As I write this, I haven't yet been blessed to be a parent, but it's been my observation as an uncle and as someone who works with kids that most parents do a terrific job instilling in their children proper values, manners, and a sense of right and wrong. But do they make the same effort when it comes to teaching their kids the Core Fundamentals of Nutrition (as well as Mindset, Movement, and Recovery)? My sense is no, if only because they've lost sight of these fundamentals themselves, or perhaps never learned them.

Kids soak up everything around them. I'm amazed at how the marketing messages targeted to adults, especially women, trickle down to girls. Girls come to believe that they shouldn't eat carbs, fats, or whatever else is part of the latest fad program. As early as the age of five, girls are establishing these eating habits. As adults we have to be cognizant of the relationship children have with food based on the messages they're receiving.

When girls reach high-school age, they enter a culture that's even more dysfunctional. They're now even more influenced by the media and the latest trends by movie stars that are just fads. They're getting their information from peers and social networks via MySpace and Facebook, and while the Internet is the greatest informational tool ever created, it's not always providing the right information, or even accurate information, when it comes to nutrition and lifestyle choices.

The reason parents work so hard to instill the proper values and morals in their children is so they will make the right choices when confronted with pressures from their peer group. So we talk to our kids about sex and drugs. But do we talk to them about proper nutrition? It might not seem as pressing a topic as sex and drugs, but not following a proper nutrition program has the potential to cause some serious long-term damage.

Perhaps the biggest tragedy of the so-called obesity epidemic is the impact it

CORE WOMEN SUCCESS STORY

"Start slow and make yourself go."

Louise Falsone • **Age: Sixty-six** • **Hometown: Buffalo, New York**

Like a lot of women in her sixties, Louise Falsone reached a turning point. Either she could continue on a downward spiral of health or she could develop a game plan for active living into her senior years.

Admittedly, it was a challenge. When her husband, Tony, died in 2004 after a long illness, she felt too emotionally spent to embark on a new lifestyle change, even though she knew it would help with her developing heart issues.

It was three years before she embarked upon the Core Performance program that her daughter had presented her.

"I really put my mind to it, realizing that it was now or never," Falsone says. "I was tired of looking like a matron. I have friends my age on the heavy side who can barely walk

because of arthritis, and they don't always see how that contributes to how you feel as an older person."

Stress had taken its toll, both in caring for her husband and also on the job, where she works at a school for developmentally delayed children. "Stress puts a lot of demands on your body that you don't realize," she says.

Living in the cold temperatures of Buffalo makes embracing a new training regimen a challenge, especially since Falsone is not a skier. Through her health plan at work, she had access to an aquatic center and a gym, where she began following the Core Performance program. When the temperatures were warm enough, she began bicycling outdoors, working her way up to rides of fifteen to twenty miles.

"If you focus not on your limitations but

on what you *can* do, you'll find that you get stronger and can do even more," Falsone says. "When I was first on the stationary bike, I thought I wouldn't be able to get through ten minutes. But you keep working at it and get back on if you have to stop. There's a psychological aspect to this, where you realize that you *can* do this. No matter what your age, you can be as healthy and mobile as you can."

Falsone also became more conscious of what she eats. That nutrition plan, along with training five to six days weekly with the Core Performance movement program, helped her to lose thirty pounds over the course of a year. The key, Falsone says, is that the program proceeded at the proper pace, even for someone in their sixties.

"Mark's program taught me to do it the right way, to make sure you're challenging yourself without pushing yourself to the limit," she says. "Someone my age is more apt to overdo it. But I found this program allows you to start slow and then make yourself go."

Falsone says she has no immediate plans to retire and is ready to face the aortic valve replacement procedure she'll need at some point. "My goal is to be as healthy as I can be so the recovery time won't be as traumatic," she says.

Nearly five years after losing her husband, she feels ready to embrace the next stages of life.

"The feelings you have for someone never go away," she says. "They're always there. But it's something where you can go forward—you can't go backward—and it took me a long time to come to that realization. I realized, 'I'm sixty-five. I have some health issues. But I know the program and I'm fully capable of doing it.'"

has on children. If parents are obese, the kids likely will be as well since they're following the same destructive eating habits and (lack of) movement patterns as their parents.

Young adult women leave home for college or the workforce armed with what parents have done to instill accountability and responsibility. That's their foundation for success. But if they leave without knowing how to assemble a nutritious meal or the importance of rest and recovery, that's almost as dangerous as not being educated about sex, alcohol, and drugs.

In college students rely on peer groups for strategies to get through the day, and it's very easy to be pulled off task even for the most grounded kids. If they don't have that instilled, they'll get spun around and struggle during that period. It's a challenging time, between the demands of class and social schedules and peer influences. They're fueling themselves and meeting the demands of life and school on their own, and if they lack these Core Fundamentals, that's a recipe for disaster.

It doesn't have to be that way. Most women are driven to succeed. They have a vision for what they want in terms of career, significant other, and family. They usually have game plans, even informal ones, for how they are going to fulfill this vision.

But whether it's fueling their bodies or those of the ones they love, that priority sometimes ends up on the back burner. Caffeine, sugar, and nutrient-bankrupt foods end up filling the energy deficit.

It's time to stop operating from a position of weakness. Rather than relying on the triple threat of sugar, caffeine, and nutrient-poor foods, we're going to only consume foods that will fuel us well, provide energy, and contribute to long-term health.

If you think that sounds like a diet, you're going to be pleasantly surprised in the next chapter.

CHAPTER 3 SUMMARY: In the last decade cultural changes have greatly impacted the way people eat. Caffeine, sugar, and foods low in nutrients and fiber play a much more prominent role, contributing to the obesity epidemic and the daily "energy crisis," where students, workers, and parents struggle to find the energy just to get through the day. The Core Performance nutrition program helps break this addiction by prescribing a balanced plan of nutrients for optimal energy.

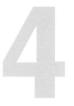

THE CORE PERFORMANCE "NON-DIET"

*di-et. noun. a: food and drink regularly provided
or consumed; b: habitual nourishment.*

'm not a fan of the word *diet*. It has such a negative connotation. We think of diet in terms of deprivation and sacrifice; indeed, the first three letters of the word are d-i-e. Nobody wants to be on a diet, which is at best a short-term solution to weight loss and no way to foster long-term health and a high-performance lifestyle.

But if we take a closer look, we find that *diet* was never intended to refer to starvation and attempted weight loss. Open the dictionary and you'll find the first two definitions of *diet* refer to "habitual nourishment." That's the key to any successful nutrition plan, identifying and *habitually* consuming the foods that *nourish* your body to give you the fuel you need to meet the challenges of daily life and *perform* as well as you possibly can.

The difference between world-class performers and those who perform well only on occasion is "habitual excellence." The world-class folks show habitual excellence. With nutrition we want to aim for world-class habitual nourishment.

Performance is the key. So many diets strip away pounds, albeit usually temporarily, and leave you starving, tired, and feeling run-down. Maybe you'll look better, though you've sacrificed your health and probably even the lean muscle mass that's the engine behind a fast metabolism. And perhaps you're even able to draw some correlation between how you look in the mirror and how it makes you feel emotionally.

"If I look good, I feel good," you try to convince yourself, as you wonder how much longer your willpower will hold you to the diet.

Unfortunately you won't be feeling good physically, since most diets require you to eliminate or greatly restrict carbohydrates and fats, two vital nutrients, or consume a ridiculous combination of foods that is not sustainable for any length of time. Research shows that most diets create a yo-yo effect; you regain the weight (and sometimes gain more) and further damage your health. The power of the Core Performance nutrition program or "non-diet" is that we take a balanced approach to nutrients that will leave you feeling energized, more productive, and, yes, happy with the way you appear in the mirror.

The difference is that you need not see your reflection to feel this way. When you have that energy and can perform better, you naturally feel better. When you're able to make the correlation between how foods affect your body and energy levels, you'll naturally gravitate toward them. You will stop dieting and start eating.

Not surprisingly, these are the same foods that when combined with even modest levels of exercise will produce a lean, powerful physique and promote long-term health. We've stripped away all of the fads, gimmicks, and mythology of conventional diet plans and left you with only the core essentials.

Best of all, this habitual nourishment need not consist of bland foods, extreme nutrient combinations of proteins, carbohydrates, and fats, or elaborate recipes that require time and vast culinary skill. Instead Core Performance nutrition consists of healthy, nourishing, and (mostly) whole foods that reflect your tastes and lifestyle.

Diet books typically give you a one-size-fits-all solution, figuring that what works for one person can be applied to everyone. But what these prescriptions overlook is that we come to the table with different habits, emotions, and associations with food that must first be addressed.

I work with women from all walks of life, including overscheduled executives, stay-at-home moms, blue-collar workers, retirees, teenagers, professional athletes, and everyone in between. Each group faces different challenges and has different nutritional needs.

One of the major fallacies of diets is their all-or-nothing approach. It's unrealistic to assume you're going to stick 100 percent to a nutrition program, even this one. Several popular diets give you a "free day" once a week to eat whatever you want, either for one meal or the entire day. Indeed, in the original *Core Performance* book, we prescribed just that. We recommended that it be Sunday, since traditionally it's a day of rest for many people, a day when they don't even train.

Since the publication of that book, however, the distinction between work and rest has been further blurred. More people seem to work on Sundays, struggling to detach from e-mail and their cell phones. When we wrote *Core Performance* books for endurance athletes and golfers, we were reminded that Sunday typically is a very active day for those folks, one in which they need high-performance fuel.

But it wasn't just an issue of Sunday or any other single day. Schedules are fluid, now more than ever, and while one of the cornerstones of our nutrition program is planning to fuel properly while on the go, on the road, and at work, life can get in the way. That's why we prescribe an 80/20 program. You're going to eat right at least 80 percent of the time and not beat yourself up about the other 20 percent of the time.

The Female Athlete Triad

BY AMANDA CARLSON, MS, RD, CSSD

By following the Core Performance for Women nutrition plan, your body will become lean and efficient. After all, excess body fat hinders performance and quality of life.

That said, there's a fine line to walk between being lean and efficient and becoming *too* lean. With women, especially those in their late teens and early twenties, we sometimes see what's known as the "female athlete triad," an obsession with body weight to the point where it becomes dangerous and leads to serious health problems.

The female athlete triad is a three-part progression, from disordered eating to amenorrhea to osteoporosis: A woman restricts calories to reduce body fat to the point where she becomes "amenorrheic"—she stops menstruating.

There's a dangerous notion that losing a normal menstrual period for only a short time is acceptable. In truth the loss of a normal menstrual period means that the body is severely out of balance.

These young women come to believe that the leaner they are, the better they will look. Therefore they start to seriously restrict their caloric intake and slip into patterns of disordered

This isn't a dramatic departure from the one-day-off approach. Eating "clean" six out of seven days represents 85.7 percent of the time. That's still a good target, but 80 percent is an acceptable benchmark.

But make no mistake; we do not mean to lower the bar. This is not a relaxed, laissez-faire approach to nutrition. Instead it's a program of *mindful* eating as opposed to the typical *mindless* consumption of food.

The difference with Core Performance nutrition is that we're not going to prescribe certain foods and dictate a set number of calories solely for the sake of weight loss. Instead we're going to help you identify the number of calories per day you need based on your nutritional goals.

eating or even a full-blown eating disorder. There are instances of women running fifteen miles a day on just 1,500 calories thinking they're eating enough.

If you restrict caloric intake too much, your performance will suffer. What these young women might perceive as a few extra calories that could boost body fat actually may help their performance and improve their energy levels and appearance.

We want to give you the solutions to stay lean, be in great health, and perform at a high level. You can have it all. So many women don't realize the damage they're doing to their bodies.

We've seen bone scans on women who have become so lean that they're showing signs of osteoporosis at the age of thirty. Their bodies no longer adapt to the demands of training. Instead they get into a downward spiral of injury and illness. All this is in addition to the long-term health consequences of early-onset osteoporosis and reduced fertility. Women in their twenties often don't consider these long-term repercussions, which in reality are not that far off.

When it comes to nutrition, listen to your body and provide it with the fuel it needs to live, train, and thrive. What you might perceive as a few extra pounds actually can help performance and ensure good health in the future.

Amanda Carlson, MS, RD, CSSD, is Director of Performance Nutrition for Athletes' Performance.

From there we'll show you how to portion these calories over the course of five or six small daily meals. For all of the nutrition books that have been written, few if any actually show you what constitutes, say, a 300-calorie meal. I don't want you obsessing over calorie counting, but I do want you to have a general idea about how many calories you're consuming.

Most important, we're going to pack as much fiber and nutrients as possible into those calories. I'm sure you've heard of the term "empty calories," foods or beverages that provide you with nothing in terms of nutrients and satiety. The opposite of this is what I call "nutrient density." We want to choose foods and create meals that pack as many nutrients as possible into the calories you consume.

In every other aspect of your life, you strive for density. You want to pack as much as possible into what limited time you have, whether it's a day, month, year, vacation, or lifetime. Why settle for anything less with your food?

Admittedly it's a challenge to cut through all of the marketing clutter, conflicting research, and downright misleading information when it comes to nutrition and food.

I spent my undergraduate and graduate years in the world of nutrition and have dedicated my career to performance coaching, and yet even I get confused. I'm befuddled by the countless diets, fads, and gimmicks out there. Some tell me not to eat carbohydrates, others no fat. I can eat certain foods, but only at certain times or during certain periods. Our heads are all spinning from the amount of marketing that is out there, pulling us in different directions, offering conflicting prescriptions.

You'd think that with this vast reservoir of "expertise" out there, the United States would have become the fittest country in the world by now. With each new diet people would be able to raise their health and fitness levels even further. Instead we've never had higher rates of obesity, diabetes, and an overall lack of health.

Never before have we been so overprogrammed and overscheduled, whether you're an executive dealing with travel and stress and the pace of business that seems to get faster every day or a stay-at-home mom dealing with the Herculean challenges of children and managing a household. Technology has allowed us to be more productive and efficient, and yet we're more exhausted and less fit.

Against this backdrop it's no wonder we search for quick-fix, efficient solutions, and indeed many of these best-selling diets provide just that. Unfortunately, by focusing on the deprivation definition of *diet*, these programs are not sustainable. Eventually you get hungry and return to your previous eating habits.

But if we concentrate on *habitual* eating patterns and the quality of the nutrients we consume on a daily basis, we can establish sustainable patterns of nourishing our bodies for optimum performance. This notion has been the cornerstone of the Core Performance program since the publication of our first book.

That book revolutionized how people train. No longer do they follow traditional bodybuilding programs of working "body parts"; they have come to understand that it's far more beneficial to train body *movements* that mimic everyday life. Just as the elite athletes I have worked with discovered that the program prevents injury and makes them more powerful, the rest of us competing in the "game of life" use the system to strengthen the shoulder, torso, and hip areas to make ourselves more resistant to injury and long-term deterioration. And, of course, we get a lean physique as a bonus.

Unfortunately the overwhelming response to the training, or Movement, portion of the book overshadowed the groundbreaking Nutrition strategies we provided. Many trainers and nutritionists, some representing professional sports teams, have found our Nutrition section more relevant and effective than anything else they've encountered.

Even readers of our books targeted to a sport-specific lifestyle audience, including *Core Performance Endurance* and *Core Performance Golf*, have said that the nutrition program has provided them the most dramatic results in terms of achieving sustainable energy and better time management.

Perhaps if we had called that first book "The Core Performance Diet," we would have attracted more readers, at least those who associate diet with the quick fix solutions typical of such books. Instead we're now able to take the Nutrition portion of our program and give it the bigger, broader platform it deserves, with the benefit of all of the research on nutrition and performance we've conducted at Athletes' Performance since the first book was written.

We also are able to incorporate all of the feedback from the raving Core Performance fans that make up our online community at www.coreperformance.com. We've taken what they've told us is most relevant and effective to driving their success and we've packaged it into an efficient system that can stand on its own in this section.

In this section we're going to reclaim the true definition of diet as "habitual intake." Until you can understand what's driving your habitual intake, the emotions, cues, and patterns, it's very difficult to make lasting change.

Think of this "non-diet" as where you draw a line in the sand and say, "Enough is enough." I've seen far too many ads for diet pills, energy drinks, instant fat-loss potions, and liposuction. All of these short-term fixes ignore what's inherently wrong. People lack the mindset and the ability to deliver quality nutrients that sustain their bodies for optimum performance.

Most of us have made the commitment to save the planet and do what we can to stop global warming. We recycle, switch to ethanol, and reduce heating and energy costs. All of this is admirable and necessary, but why is it we can't take the same approach when it comes to saving our bodies and our health? None of us can save the planet—we can do our part—but the one thing we can control is what goes into our mouths.

So many people dig their own graves with a fork and spoon and the "dirt" they're shoveling into their mouths. The next time you're grocery shopping, keep your head down and stare only at the contents of shopping carts. Then steal a glance at the people pushing them. You'll find that their appearance, from weight and body composition to skin tone and hair, is directly proportionate to what they have in their carts.

Most people recognize the high cost of smoking. Set aside for a moment the health and lifestyle costs; smoking is *literally* expensive. But people rarely consider the financial costs of eating poorly. They usually understand the health risks, though they're often fooled by marketing and misleading food labels, but they fail to recognize that this lifestyle of eating out frequently and consuming a lot of processed junk is more expensive than following a high-performance nutrition plan.

Like smokers, these people are paying a premium to inflict harm on their bodies!

We have an obesity crisis because we haven't been honest with ourselves. We think it's all about fixing the problem through dieting. If you blow out a tire because your wheel is not aligned properly, a new tire is only a short-term solution. Likewise, if you think a diet is going to solve a habitual intake of poor food grounded in an improper mindset, you're fooling yourself.

It's time to provide a simple, clear, honest plan that cuts through the fad diets and says here is what you need to do—and why. Here is how you've conditioned your mind to think and here's how we can untangle the wiring and get you back on track. Most important, this will be an easy-to-follow, personalized nutrition plan that can help you not just survive but *thrive* in your hectic lifestyle.

One of the best things you can do to improve your health is to become an educated consumer. Whether ordering a restaurant meal or reading an ingredients label, you need to make the best decision for your healthy lifestyle.

You must also plan and prepare. Otherwise you're at the mercy of what's out there, and most of it isn't good. The most common reason people eat improperly and sabotage their nutrition program is shoddy planning.

When it comes to nutrition, like everything else in this program, you have to think long-term. It's easy to rationalize eating unhealthy food—after all, you're hungry and you need to eat something. You're not *that* overweight. You haven't eaten all day. You are stressed, tired, and you deserve it. Perhaps you don't want to be rude to your hosts or just want to eat what your kids or significant other is having. Maybe you're not overweight at all and feel free to eat as much or as little as you like.

It is very easy to fall down the slippery slope of excuses when it comes to putting food into our mouths. Remember, those few moments of pleasure junk food provides end quickly. So, too, does the value of the food in terms of producing energy. Soon you'll be hungry again, further contributing to the negative long-term impact that unhealthy food has on your body and your mind.

Make a positive investment instead. Each time you eat properly, remind yourself that you're not only giving yourself the energy needed for optimal performance, but you're also investing in your long-term health—to say nothing of helping yourself look, feel, and perform better. The reason most diet plans fail is that they tend to address the symptoms—too much weight and lack of energy—rather than the problem, which is poor nutrition in general. You're not fueling your life properly.

Stressing out over where and when to eat is unhealthy, a problem made worse by the junk you inevitably consume in such a state. As a result, you end up adding body fat and losing lean mass, which defeats the purpose of following the rest of the Core Performance for Women program. Not only that, but eating on the run is expensive and compromises your health.

In the next chapter we're going to examine the Mindset behind Nutrition and help you understand the emotions guiding your food choices. For now, let's dispel some popular misconceptions about proper nutrition.

Eating right means you'll eat only bland, tasteless food. This is a big misconception. It's easy to prepare meals that are full of color, healthy, and, most important, tasty. There are dozens of delicious foods, condiments, and spices that will help you to eat meals that are as delicious as they are good for you.

Fast-food restaurants thrive because they perpetuate these myths. Habitual intake of such "food" conditions your brain to believe that this processed junk actually tastes good. In the movie *Super Size Me*, filmmaker Morgan Spurlock attempted to eat nothing but McDonald's food for a month. The more he ate, the more he craved it, even as his health grew worse and his energy levels plummeted.

Once you're able to make the connection between how healthy food can make you feel better, you'll start to crave it. Low-nutrient foods, whether high-sugar or sugar-free, high in fat or fat-free, rob you of energy, produce nasty mood swings, and increase body fat. Again, healthy food need not be tasteless chow. In this section you'll discover many foods to mix and match for tasty meals and snacks.

Eating right is expensive. Actually, eating right saves money. If you've planned your day and week, chances are you'll eat out infrequently, which saves a lot of cash. When you have not prepared ahead of time you're more likely to grab the first option available. Not only is that likely to be unhealthy, it probably will be expensive.

Think of how often you grabbed food on the go or ordered takeout simply because you knew there was nothing at home. Granted, you could go for some nutritious options on the run—and we'll show you how to make those choices—but that's an expensive way to eat for the long haul.

Eating right is time-consuming. On the contrary, eating right saves time. If you have your meals plotted out for the entire day—or the entire week—you'll save hours each week. Let's compare a woman who brings her lunch to work with one who has to go get takeout. The one who brought lunch already has saved a minimum of fifteen to thirty minutes, and it's more likely she'll eat a more healthful alternative. Not only that, but if you have lunch handy, you're less likely to go hungry and rush out to find the first option available, which usually is a losing battle.

It's not necessary to eat at your desk, though some women in the corporate world find that eating there frees up enough time over lunch hour to work out, especially if there's a gym on-site.

One easy way to get a jump start on the week is to do all of your shopping on Saturdays or Sundays, which will help you plan meals for the week. This is a great way to be proactive about your choices. I guarantee that a little planning, preparing, and organization of your environment will get you looking and feeling the way you want.

It's time to stop viewing food as the enemy. Instead look at it as one of your closest allies in the fight against disease, fatigue, inflammation, and injury. View nutrition as your workout partner, an essential tool to optimize your health, training, and performance.

So many women view food either with fear ("It will make me fat") or with love ("I live to eat"). Make an effort not to fear your food or obsess over it. Instead you should eat to live—look at food objectively, as a potentially powerful means to fuel your performance.

If you take nothing away from the Nutrition section of this program, remember this: Starving yourself and going hungry will make you fat. That's right. In the short term, you

CORE WOMEN SUCCESS STORY

"People ask if I had gastric bypass surgery."

Mary Iverson • **Age: Forty-six** • **Hometown: Detroit, Michigan**

Mary Iverson grew up with no nutrition rules. Her diet was mostly sugary cereals, cake, and prepackaged snack foods. The only vegetables she consumed were starchy ones like potatoes and corn. She was in her forties before she ate a salad.

"I'm the fourth of five children," she says. "I think by the time my little brother and I came along, Mom just gave up and let us all eat whatever."

Like many overweight children of her generation, she remembers the humiliation of not getting picked for sports teams. "I was the fat kid nobody wanted," she says.

Iverson managed to lose weight in high school by limiting herself to just one meal a day. Some days that was a bowl of Cheerios. She joined the track-and-field team, competing as a shot-putter, and kept the weight off through her starvation diet.

As a working adult, she packed on ten to twenty pounds a year, eventually ballooning to 240 pounds on her 5-foot-2 frame. She struggled to find size 26 clothes, buying shirts sized XXXL and meant for men.

Iverson's mother and two brothers are morbidly obese and another brother is overweight. Mom and a brother suffer from heart disease, a direct result of their eating habits and lack of activity. Her paternal grandmother, a squatty woman almost as wide around as she was tall, died at fifty.

Iverson remembers seeing pictures of her mother as a slender young lady, a stark contrast to the obese older woman confined to the sofa and bed by type-2 diabetes. She envisioned a similar future for herself if she did not change.

"It really is true that if you have your health you have everything," Iverson says. "You rush around and you forget sometimes how great it is to be able just to move. Then I'll look at my mom and how she can't walk and what that's done to her."

By following the Core Performance program over several years, Iverson dropped ninety pounds and shrunk from a size 26 to a 10. Instead of engaging in random cardio activities that did little to create lean muscle, she dedicated herself to the Movement portion of the program. But it was the Nutrition component that required more dramatic change.

Iverson learned to eat and even enjoy salads. She discovered she preferred spinach because of its rich taste. Instead of ordering typical restaurant portions, she requests kid's meals. She remains a chocoholic, but now chocolate is a much-earned treat and not a dietary staple.

"I'll still walk through the diet section of bookstores and see all of these programs that just aren't realistic," she says. "I feel that the Core Performance diet is more sustainable."

For years Iverson thought nothing of consuming a large bag of snack chips or an entire bag of cookies in one sitting. She says the key to her weight loss was identifying her emotional eating habits and understanding that the so-called comfort food was anything but.

"Now when I eat snack food I feel sick," she says.

These days Iverson glances in the mirror and wonders who the person staring back is. Her husband notes that she no longer huffs and puffs as she climbs the stairs to their third-floor home. So dramatic is the change that people have asked her if she underwent gastric bypass surgery.

Iverson recently gained more than five pounds as a result of some medication and made it clear to the doctor that such side effects were unacceptable.

"I will not go back to where I was," she says. "My only regret is that I waited so long to make the journey to a healthier lifestyle."

might lose some weight, though you'll feel miserable in the process. When you don't give your body the fuel it needs, it becomes catabolic, drawing fuel from and depleting your lean muscle—the very thing you've worked so hard to create. It's this lean muscle or "lean mass" that burns calories at a greater rate, even when you're resting. Unfortunately this is the first thing your body turns to for fuel in this catabolic state.

When your body lacks the proper fuel to run or recover, its ability to take on the stress of daily life and training is substantially compromised, and it never has a chance to fully heal. This unbalanced state makes you more susceptible to sickness, fatigue, depression, inflammation, injury, and loss of motivation.

Even if you think you're eating properly right now, I guarantee that the following pages will show you ways to eat better and improve performance. Nutrition should be used to enhance your health, your energy, and your performance in everything that you do.

CHAPTER 4 SUMMARY: Those who follow traditional weight-loss diets are doomed to fail, since such programs do not provide adequate calories and a proper balance of nutrients. Core Performance Women nutrition is a "non-diet" because there's no deprivation, just proper fuel for your hectic life. By following this simple plan, you'll have more energy while saving time and money, discovering tasty, nutritious food along the way.

FOOD IS NOT THE ENEMY

ake a moment and consider how you eat. Do you eat large quanti-
ties of food or poor-quality food when you get stressed, get inadequate sleep, during relationship troubles, or when you're having
perhaps a bit too much fun? Do you eat differently when you travel?

Anyone who has tried to stop smoking understands the idea of triggers. In order to quit smoking it's necessary to stop linking cigarettes to
certain behaviors such as driving, while drinking, after meals, and after
sex. Unlike cigarettes, the goal with food is not to stop completely; we
must continue eating.

Food presents a different set of triggers. It's possible to eat and feel
full but not be nourished when your body doesn't get the right nutrients.

Core Performance Habit Screen

A. Yes! How did you know this was me?

B. I guess I feel like this sometimes, maybe most of the time.

C. Nope, not me at all.

____ 1. When I eat a "bad" food, I feel guilty and that I have cheated.

____ 2. Food is comforting to me.

____ 3. I tend to eat whatever is around and convenient rather than plan my meals.

____ 4. I feel that I spend a lot of time thinking about my body and weight and less time actually working toward my goal.

____ 5. I eat most of my food after five p.m.

____ 6. I struggle between foods that I know I should eat and foods that I *want* to eat.

____ 7. If I am trying to lose weight, skipping meals or severely cutting back calories is my strategy.

____ 8. My weight and body are a major source of frustration. At some point I have even cried about my weight.

____ 9. I don't really understand what portions are right for me and my goals.

So what happens? Your body doesn't perform well, even though you don't feel hungry. Still, you reach for something to fill the void, often the same low-quality foods you had earlier.

You need to understand what's going on in your head. What goes on between your ears is what's opening the lever to your jaw. So if we better understand that thinking, then we can understand why we're reaching for things, whether positive or negative. As soon as you make that connection, you have the foundation for what you need to make lasting change.

___ 10. When I am under stress, anxious, lonely, tired, or depressed, I tend to eat differently—typically worse.

___ 11. I find myself eating very little during the day. By the time the evening hits, I am starving.

___ 12. I tend not to plan my meals. I just eat whatever is available.

___ 13. I know I need to change my nutritional habits, but I can't seem to get started.

___ 14. I eat differently when I am alone than when I am around other people.

___ 15. When I am busy I tend to skip meals or forget to eat.

___ 16. I let my emotions be an excuse for changing the way I eat.

___ 17. I tend to overeat when there is no limit to the food available.

___ 18. I always seem to wait till the last minute to start a project.

___ 19. I feel like I am constantly eating between dinner and bedtime. I think I eat most of my food during that period of time.

___ 20. I don't have consistent meal patterns from one day to another. Each day is different.

___ 21. When I make dinner at home, I tend to snack on food while cooking.

Please take a moment to answer the questionnaire above. Be honest with yourself as you take the test, answering the way you live right now, not the way you hope to approach food or the way you presume is correct. Read each statement and choose one of the three answers A, B, or C.

If you answered A or B frequently, you've developed a lot of bad eating habits, letting emotions and inconsistent energy levels dictate how you eat. Don't worry. Through this program, you'll learn to be more proactive with your eating and better control your energy levels and thus your emotions. Keep the results of this survey and take it again after a few months. You'll likely get much different results.

We have found that there are five eating styles or behaviors that typically derail the best intentions women have to follow a good nutrition program. They are The Procrastinator, The Emotional Eater, The Reactive Eater, The Portion Distortionist, and The Evening Eater. Women who answer "A" or "B" frequently tend to fall into one or more of these categories. Let's take a look at each category and examine how to change the mindset of each.

The Procrastinator

It's difficult to embark on a new nutritional program. It's easy to maintain the status quo.

The Procrastinator knows that it's time to make a change. She wants to make a change but continuously comes up with excuses to avoid it. There is always something that is getting in the way of getting started. Whether it is a family responsibility, a weekend party, work deadline, or the holiday season, the Procrastinator never seems to get started on a new way of eating. She puts it off until after the weekend or the holidays or until life slows down.

Of course life never slows down. The tentative start date comes and goes. You keep finding reasons not to start a new plan. It's a destructive habit. By putting things off, you probably do not get started on things early enough and find yourself crunching at a deadline. Whether it is cleaning the house, organizing a closet, or starting a new work project, you never seem to get it started when you want.

Many women want to have a strong "internal feeling" that pushes them into getting started; however, that push rarely comes. The longer you wait to start a new way of eating (or training regimen), the longer your health and condition will continue to deteriorate. Everyone procrastinates at some time or another, but if it is affecting your health, weight, or livelihood, there is no time like the present to spring into action.

How to Cook and Bake in a Healthier Way

- Preserve nutrients and color in veggies by steaming or stir-frying. Don't boil veggies.

- Use vegetable spray or nonstick pans for stir-frying and sautéing.

- Find ways to sneak in veggies, such as adding carrot and sweet potato puree to tomato sauces. You also can add shredded carrots and potatoes to meatloaf and hamburgers to reduce the amount of meat.

- Keep open-flame grilling to a minimum. Charred foods contain cancer-promoting compounds.

- When following recipes, cut the salt in half. There won't be a noticeable change.

- Use evaporated skim milk in place of cream or half-and-half.

- Increase your fiber intake by sprinkling in wheat bran flakes and ground flaxseed when cooking and baking.

- Reduce the fat in baked goods by substituting mashed bananas, applesauce, or yogurt for up to half of the butter or shortening in the recipe.

- Substitute whole-wheat flour for all-purpose flour in your cooking. Whole-wheat flour can be substituted for up to half of the all-purpose flour.

- Make fruit desserts instead of cakes and cookies. Choose frozen yogurt, sherbet, and sorbet instead of ice cream.

- Use sensible cooking techniques with less fat and add more vegetables, fruits, and whole grains to recipes to increase the nutritional value of your meals, snacks, and desserts.

If following a new nutrition program seems daunting, set yourself up for success by taking small steps. Print your grocery list at the beginning of the week and place a copy on the fridge. Keep fresh fruit and healthy snacks at home, in your office, and in your bag. Keep a water bottle with you at all times to remind yourself to drink water regularly. Clear out the fridge and pantry and restock with healthy food.

By breaking your large goal up into more manageable pieces, you will set yourself up for success and give yourself a road map of checkpoints along the way to the end of your goal, which is a new, healthy habit.

Celebrate little victories, whether it's skipping the fast-food drive-thru to make a healthy dinner at home or simply eating healthy snacks throughout the day. Recognize that there will be times when you fall off the wagon. When that happens, don't beat yourself up over it. Just get right back on the program. Great nutrition, increased energy, and a lean physique do not come from a few actions; they come from the sum of those actions that happen over the long haul.

But before any of this happens, you have to start somewhere. That time is now.

The Emotional Eater

Many women suffer from emotional eating. For some Emotional Eaters, food becomes a source of comfort during times of stress, anxiety, sadness, loneliness, boredom, depression, or even in times of celebration. The Emotional Eater turns to eating as a way to make herself feel better, affirm her feelings, give her a sense that she deserves a treat, or simply to occupy herself during lonely times.

During these emotional situations she finds herself drawn to certain foods; they even become a reward. After a long, stressful week at work or after an emotionally draining argument with a friend or spouse, she finds herself believing that she's "earned" her favorite comfort food. Eating to soothe emotions often provides an immediate feeling of relief. After she indulges herself, she often feels happy or satisfied. Unfortunately these feelings are short-term, and she's left feeling guilty, ashamed, and defeated. This could quickly turn into a downward spiral that compromises her self-esteem and sabotages the potential for a healthier lifestyle.

For other Emotional Eaters, food becomes the enemy, something to avoid or restrict in times of stress. This type of Emotional Eater may find herself having an internal struggle between eating in general—healthy food or not-so-healthy treats. She finds a sense of control in not eating or restricting her intake. This leads to moodiness, low energy, and eventually hunger that no longer can be ignored. At that point, when the hunger is so great, good choices are rarely made; she often overeats. The cycle begins again: restrict, binge, feel guilt. Restrict, binge, feel guilt.

The problem with emotional eating is that every day presents new stresses, anxieties, and problems. By continually using food as a coping mechanism, you're apt to rely on it to soothe feelings. When you consistently use food as a response to an emotion you're feeling, you are sabotaging your own efforts to create new, healthy habits. During emotional eating you often choose the wrong food and eat too much of it. Few people will run to the refrigerator for chopped vegetables and hummus after a tough day at work. Perhaps you've started on the road to achieving the goals you've defined for a new, healthy lifestyle, but your emotional eating is slowing down your progress. This prevents you from fully reaping the benefits of your effort, leaving you discouraged and unmotivated.

To combat your emotional eating, it's necessary to recognize the feelings and situations that serve as triggers. Next you must find ways to deal with these emotions other than with food. Be patient. Creating new habits takes time. Figuring out why you are eating the food you are eating and dealing with those emotions head-on will help you to experience freedom from the destructive habit of emotional eating.

One of the best ways to tackle emotional eating is to keep a diary to track your mood when you're eating. This will help link your mood to certain types of food. As you jot down the food that you are eating, record what situation occurred before you ate and how you were feeling at the time. By doing this you will start to see connections between your emotions and certain foods. An example might include:

Got in a fight with my coworker.

Went to McDonald's and got a large fries and a Coke.

Felt entitled to eat something I enjoy but later felt guilty for eating the high-fat, high-sugar meal.

The key to dealing with emotional eating is to identify your eating trends and emotional triggers. Once that's accomplished, you can begin to put a plan in place that will help you overcome your use of food as a coping mechanism during times of distress.

In this program you'll discover that you're better able to deal with stress and thus avoid emotional eating. Emotions will not disappear, but by being aware of how you use food and by maintaining consistency in how you eat—preferably every two to three hours—you'll maintain blood sugar levels and avoid the wild mood swings that lead to emotional eating. Not only that, the Core Performance workout sessions will help you better deal with stress and put you in a better mindset to avoid such triggers.

Finally, and most important, the way you view eating will change. Most of the time you will eat nutrient-dense foods, always conscious of how they impact your body. You might still have the occasional emotional meal or snack, but this no longer will derail your habitual intake or your mental state.

The Reactive Eater

For the Reactive Eater, there is little structure to eating and a lack of awareness of the amount of food consumed over the course of the day. This sporadic, reactive approach to nutrition can make it seem difficult to change, but once you are aware of your actions, it's actually quite easy.

As with many aspects of life, structure is the key to success. When we have structure, we're more likely to follow through; in this way habits are formed. So many people plot their days and goals down to the most trivial details. Everything, it seems, is scheduled.

Unfortunately, food and nutrition usually are not part of such extensive to-do lists. Meals (and workouts) don't make it into the day planner. This creates an environment that sets the stage for reactive eating.

The Reactive Eater eats in the car, grabs calories from vending machines, or swings through fast-food restaurants or finds herself so wrapped up in work and life that she just forgets to eat. This eating style leads to missed meals, which further exacerbates the problem. It's no wonder you are ready to grab whatever is closest to calm your hunger. Instead, we want to be proactive about what we're eating. This will eliminate those missed meals, those hunger pangs, and even decrease your likelihood to give in to food that may throw you off of your healthy nutrition plan.

If you eat while doing other things, you might not be in tune with your hunger. You might be making choices based on what is most convenient rather than what is best for your needs. If you don't plan meals, you might be unaware of what or how much of what it is that you really do eat.

Instead of being Reactive Eaters, we want to be *proactive* eaters, planning our meals to save time and money and fuel our success. A proactive eater is far more likely to make healthy choices and less likely to skip meals. A proactive eater also will eat more high-nutrient, energy-producing foods.

Be mindful of when you're eating and where. Turn off the television, get out of the car, and step away from your desk. Give yourself time to eat. All too often we eat while doing other things and we don't really think about how much we are eating or why we are eating it.

Keeping a food journal is another excellent way to avoid reactive eating. Log the time you eat, what you eat, how much you eat, how hungry you were, and where you ate (desk, cafeteria, etc.). Track a couple days a week each week to help you get acquainted with this new type of eating.

As part of your journal, plan your meals for the upcoming week and then shop for and prepare them. This need not be implemented for all seven days immediately. Aim for planning for three days the first week, four the second, and five the third week. Just as it's necessary to plan and set goals for other aspects of life, it's important to plan meals in order to have success with nutrition. I can't overstate the importance of journaling. Financial planners often ask new clients to chronicle every penny they spend over the course of several weeks. Most people have a pretty good idea of the big-ticket items—mortgage, car expenses, food, utility and phone bills, etc.—but far underestimate their discretionary spending.

The same is true with food. You might only be thinking in terms of what you eat for breakfast, lunch, and dinner. But when you see on paper all of your "discretionary eating" and what prompted it, it's an eye-opening experience. You'll likely see some vending machine and convenience store runs, late-night snacking, and all too many trips to Starbucks for high-calorie, high-sugar energy replacement.

Journaling will help you get in touch with your body and its cues of hunger and fullness. As you start to eat more frequently and in a more structured pattern, take note of your feelings of fullness and your hunger. When you skip meals, you will be hungrier at the next mealtime. You can note this in your food journal. As you begin to eat proactively and consistently, you will not be as hungry at meals and will be less likely to overeat. It's not necessary to keep a journal indefinitely, but periodically monitoring your nutritional habits is a good practice. After all, it is the sum of our habits that determine our energy levels and body composition. It's not always necessary to focus on the food itself, just the habits behind what is motivating us to put it into our mouths.

Anticipate your environment and prepare for it. If you know there are unhealthy snacks in the vending machine at work, take your own mini-meals. If there is nothing to eat after a workout, take what you need in the car. If what you need is not around, put it into your environment. You wouldn't go out in a snowstorm without boots, gloves, and a coat. Keep yourself prepared to eat as healthfully as possible all of the time. (We'll examine those nutrients in depth in the next chapter.)

Admittedly, changing habits can be difficult. But with just a little planning and some awareness of why you eat the way you do, it's possible to take inches off your body and put more stable energy in your tank.

The Portion Distortionist

The Portion Distortionist does not understand how much food her body needs. She overeats both on healthy food and junk or might restrict eating to maintain a certain weight. Such women do not know when to say when—or know when they actually need to eat more.

If you eat too much, perhaps it's because you were raised to clean your plate or just grew accustomed to eating large amounts of food. Bigger portions became a way of life at home and while eating out. You rarely cut a portion in half or even have an idea of how much you should be eating. The size of restaurant meals keeps getting bigger, and so do you.

People under the age of twenty-five have no recollection of the 8-ounce soda bottle, three-inch bagel, small french fries, or the twelve-inch pizza for four people. Theirs is the generation of the 20-ounce soda and the supersize hamburger, pizza, and fries. They don't know life without ranch dressing served with everything. Our modern environment makes it difficult to "eat small."

Just like your car has a tank to hold a certain amount of gas, your body needs only so much fuel. When your portion sizes are continually more than what you need, your tank will spill over, and this translates into additional pounds on the scale. Your continual overeating makes you more susceptible to heartburn, indigestion, or acid reflux.

Each time you overeat you promise yourself never to do it again, only to repeat the process. And each time you are left with a feeling of guilt, establishing a destructive cycle.

If you eat too little to maintain energy and performance, you're probably unaware of how many calories your body needs. Many women perceive a daily intake of 1,800 to 2,200 calories as a huge amount, but that's actually what the body needs to keep going. Calorie restrictors find that when they add the calories back—or for the first time—their energy, performance, and body composition improves. Admittedly it's counterintuitive to think that if you eat more you will lose body fat. But if you are not giving your body what it needs, it will hold on to those precious fat stores because of the fear of starving.

On the flip side, if your body is constantly running on empty or near empty, you're not as efficient. Eating becomes a constant source of stress and anxiety.

The first thing to do is to be aware of your hunger level and eating habits. Here, too, it's important to keep a food journal. For each meal and snack, record what time you eat and drink, what it is and how much of it you are consuming, how hungry you are at the time of the meal or snack, and where you are eating your meal.

By doing this you will start to see patterns emerge. You will start to identify times when you are more likely to have large portions or inadequate portions and times when portion control is no problem. After identifying the situations where portions are out of control, you can be aware and plan ahead to avoid excess consumption.

As the world has become supersized, everyone has lost touch with what a portion should be. When you write in your food journal, compare and contrast your portion sizes to that of an actual portion size. It might seem cumbersome to measure food, but it's an easy habit to establish in order to understand what a portion of our favorite foods looks like.

Once you figure out what a portion size actually is, you probably will find that you are eating two or three times the servings you need if you are trying to lose weight. A deck of cards is the size of one serving of protein, and your fist is equivalent to one serving of rice, pasta, or cooked cereal.

Imagine your plate with three sections. Half of your plate should consist of fruits and vegetables. The other half should be split between protein and whole-grain carbohydrates (whole-wheat pasta, whole-wheat couscous, whole-wheat bread, etc.). Another easy way to keep your portions in check is to use a smaller plate or bowl.

Less surface area = less eaten. When dining in restaurants, cut your meal in half and take the other half home. Decline the bread basket and ask for salad dressing on the side. If it's a buffet, make just one trip.

The Evening Eater

The Evening Eater consumes most of her calories from dinner on into the evening. Evening Eaters have very little during the day, either intentionally skipping meals or being too busy to eat, or simply they are not hungry. As evening approaches, hunger takes over and they end up feeling ravenous. Evening Eaters find themselves racing to the pantry or fridge immediately after getting home from work and overindulging on the first thing they find. Such overeating leads to feelings of guilt and being stuffed. The next day she does not feel hungry initially and later she tries not to eat much because of how much she ate the night before.

The Evening Eater gets into a destructive cycle of undereating during the day and overeating at night, creating an imbalanced eating pattern that does not include proper nutrition during the day. She has insufficient energy to deal with the daily grind, leaving her starved by dinnertime. But just as her activity level winds down, her food intake picks up. This is exactly opposite of what you need to do in order to control your weight, maintain sufficient energy, and lead a healthy lifestyle.

A little planning goes a long way. Eating throughout the day might be an adjustment, or perhaps you lack structure to your eating schedule. Here are some tips:

Put nutrition into a schedule. Think about what time you are going to eat all of your meals and snacks. Write it in your food journal, planner, and calendar. Remember: Food is fuel. Without it you will not have the energy you need to accomplish what you need to do. Make it a priority to eat your meals and snacks, eating every 2½ to 3 hours. Your intake should consist of breakfast, midmorning snack, lunch, midafternoon snack, dinner, and maybe one midevening snack.

Create an environment for success. By filling your environment with healthy options, you will be more likely to make healthy choices. Take a look in your fridge, pantry, office, briefcase, and purse. If you have unhealthy options, get rid of them. Replace these not-so-great choices with foods that will provide you with the energy and the nutrients that you need.

This task of controlling portions, developing a healthy relationship with food, and avoiding emotional, reactive eating might seem like a daunting one. Fortunately everything you need to accomplish this task and free you from these destructive habits can be summarized in four simple rules.

CHAPTER 5 SUMMARY: Women often let emotions dictate their relationship with food, which leads to overeating and consuming the wrong types of food. Typical is the Emotional Eater or Reactive Eater who does not have a nutrition plan or daily strategy but rather lets outside forces and stress dictate when, what, and even *if* she eats.

Another challenge is eating proper portions, with restaurant meals in particular providing far too much food for one sitting. By recognizing proper portion size, along with the emotional triggers and lack of planning, it's possible to get a handle on nutrition and fuel the body for optimal success. By taking time to look inward and evaluate what is driving us to eat the way we do, it's possible to make lasting positive change.

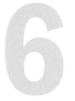

THE FOUR NEW RULES OF NUTRITION

Amanda Carlson, our Director of Performance Nutrition at Athletes' Performance, has spent her career studying nutrition. She's come up with nutrition programs for countless women, all looking to become leaner, stronger, and possess more energy. You would think that with Amanda's multiple degrees and vast expertise in the field of nutrition, she would have a lengthy, complex set of rules to follow when it comes to fueling your body.

Actually, her prescription is quite simple. That's a good thing since none of us—women or men—have the time, ability, or willingness to take the everyday task of eating and make it a chore, which is what so many diet programs force us to do.

Core Performance Women breaks nutrition down into four simple strategies, along with some advice on what to eat before, during, and after a workout. If you can master these techniques, combined with the Core Performance Women workout program, you'll be in phenomenal position to thrive in all aspects of your life.

Rule #1: Eat Clean

When it comes to eating clean, it's not just about washing your food thoroughly, though that's always important. Eating clean refers to making the best possible choice whenever you're selecting food. Amanda encourages women to "come back to earth," choosing the least-processed food available.

Whole foods are the best choice, since they're unprocessed and unrefined, or at least processed and refined as little as possible prior to consumption. Whole foods typically do not contain added salt, sugar, and fat.

When grocery shopping you'll usually find whole foods on the perimeter of the store. That's where you'll find the produce, meat and seafood, dairy, frozen foods, and other natural foods. These areas are refrigerated, which is no coincidence. The less processed a food is, the shorter the shelf life.

The middle aisles of a grocery story are the danger zone. Here you'll find snack foods, baking supplies, cereals, sodas, and condiments. Many of these processed foods can (and do) remain on shelves for months. It's not necessary to avoid these aisles altogether—there are some nutritional gems to be found, such as tea and whole-wheat pasta and couscous—but generally it's a good rule of thumb to work the perimeter.

Eating clean also means consuming the proper mix of carbs, proteins, and fats. All food is classified into these three nutrient groups, and if you neglect any of the three, you deprive your body of important nutrients you need to perform at your best.

Carbs: aka "Power Fuel"

Throughout the 1990s popular diets conditioned people to believe that carbohydrates must be avoided at all costs. Just as the anti-fat trend of the 1980s indiscriminately gave fats a bad name, carbs were unfairly labeled as the enemy. Thankfully most people now recognize the importance of carbs to healthy eating.

Carbs are our primary fuel source. They provide energy for muscle function and act as the primary fuel for the brain. When you don't take in enough carbs, your body does not run efficiently or effectively. Think of carbs as the fuel for your body's gas tank. When consumed in the proper amounts, carbs are used for energy and stored in the liver and the muscles for future energy needs. If you eat too many carbs, they will overflow the gas tank and be stored as fat. But if you don't eat enough carbs, you'll run out of fuel, which means low energy, decreased focus, and even nasty mood swings.

You need to fuel your body based on the size of your gas tank. When you follow the Core Performance Women program, you will require much more fuel than someone who doesn't exercise. Working out regularly burns a lot of fuel and demands sufficient carbs. As your training increases over the course of a week, month, or year, so should your carbohydrate intake. It's that simple: Eat carbs in *proportion* to your activity. However, don't lump yourself in with the sedentary and inactive—low carb diets are not for you, and you will start to see a decline in your energy level and performance should you follow such a program.

Not all carbs are created equal. When planning meals, avoid processed carbs such as white breads, pastas, and baked goods. They provide little nutritional value and are converted quickly to sugar and easily stored as fat.

Instead include fruits, vegetables, beans, and whole grains for their fiber and nutrient density. Your meals should consist mostly of colorful high-fiber vegetables and antioxidants that help to protect the body from the cell-damaging effects of free radi-

Fiber Up

Most people don't get nearly enough fiber in their diet; you need between 25 and 30 grams per day, and most people get less than half that amount. When choosing whole grains, look for products that include at least 3 grams of fiber per serving. Because fiber is found mostly in carbohydrates and is essential to overall health, people who follow low-carb diet plans deprive themselves of this vital source of nutrition.

Fiber improves gastrointestinal health and function and helps prevent colon cancer. It regulates blood sugar levels, keeps you full, and promotes long-term cardiovascular health by reducing cholesterol. Heart disease is the number-one killer of women. Cholesterol levels, which are correlated with heart disease, can be controlled by getting adequate fiber in your diet. Fiber is found in oatmeal, beans, whole grains, fruits, and green leafy vegetables. You can also get it in bottled form. Psyllium-based products, such as Metamucil, are a terrific source of fiber that you can sprinkle on your meals to improve their nutritional value or even mix into water and drink. Our mothers and grandmothers were not crazy when they would mix the fiber into liquid in the morning. Now we know that fiber and fiber supplements go far beyond helping our "regularity" and are vital to cardiovascular health.

cals. If you opt for pasta or couscous, choose the whole-wheat option. If you reach for rice, opt for brown rice or wild rice.

One of my favorite sayings is "Eat a rainbow often." When you look at your plate, you should see a lot of color from fruits, vegetables, and high-fiber grains.

Meal Assembly

These days it's difficult to find time to plan, prepare, and enjoy full meals. That's why I find it valuable to "assemble" meals rather than cook or prepare them.

Prepare for your week on Sunday by grilling a large quantity of chicken, fish, and lean red meat. Steam vegetables and slice tomatoes. Cook plenty of good carbs, such as sweet potatoes, brown rice, and whole-wheat couscous and pasta. Grab some prepackaged organic salad mixes and place everything into single-serving containers. That way you'll have plenty of food for the week ahead.

Another easy strategy is to purchase precooked rotisserie chickens, which are readily available and inexpensive. Peel off the skin, pat away the excess oil, cut up the bird, and you'll have enough meat for two to four single meals.

Not only will you have meals to get you through much of the workweek, but you also can fill a small cooler and keep it in the car for those weekend days when you're out training or running errands. You'll find that it's easy to create a high-performance nutrition plan that's adaptable to any lifestyle and that saves you time and money.

GRAINS/STARCHES	
PASTA/RICE	
¼ cup	risotto-quinoa (cooked)
⅓ cup	brown rice, cooked
⅓ cup	whole-wheat couscous (cooked)
½ cup	whole-wheat pasta (cooked)
BREAD/TORTILLAS/ROLLS	
1 slice	whole-wheat bread
½	pita bread (6-inch diameter)
¼	whole-wheat bagel
½	whole-wheat English muffin
½	whole-wheat hamburger roll/ hot dog bun
½	sub bread (6 inches each)
1	whole-wheat or corn tortilla (6 inches)
2	corn tortillas (4-inch diameter)
1 small	whole-wheat roll (~1 ounce)
COLD CEREALS	
½ cup	All-Bran
¾ cup	Cheerios
¾ cup	Cheerios MultiGrain
½ cup	Frosted Mini Wheats
½ cup	Grape-Nuts
½ cup	Kashi Go Lean
½ cup	Mueslix
½ cup	Raisin Bran
¾ cup	Special K
½ cup	whole-wheat Total
HOT CEREALS	
½ cup	Cream of Wheat (cooked)
1 packet	instant grits
½	packet Kashi instant oatmeal

½	packet Quaker instant oatmeal
½ cup	slow-cooked oatmeal (cooked)
VEGGIES, BEANS, POTATOES	
½ cup	cooked or canned beans
1 cup	squash (winter, acorn, butternut)
½ cup	peas (cooked)
½ small	baked potato
½ cup	corn (cooked)
1	medium ear of corn
½ cup	sweet potato (cooked)
½ cup	yam (cooked)
½ cup	lentils (cooked)
½ cup	mashed potatoes
SNACKS/CRACKERS/GRANOLA BARS	
1	Kashi granola bar
2	graham crackers
5	whole-wheat crackers (baked)
4	whole-wheat melba toast
1	Nature Valley granola bar
8	animal crackers
3 cups	light popcorn (popped)
¾ cup	pretzels
2	rice cakes (4 inches each)
1	whole-grain Fig Newton
PROTEINS	
FISH/SEAFOOD	
3 ounces	salmon, halibut, tuna, etc.
POULTRY	
3 ounces	chicken breast or lunch meat
3 ounces	ground turkey (cooked)
3 ounces	turkey breast or lunch meat

BEEF/PORK	
3 ounces	beef (96% lean ground chuck)
1½ ounces	beef jerky
3 ounces	beef tenderloin
3 ounces	London broil
3 ounces	pork (grilled)
3 ounces	roast beef (lunch meat)

DAIRY	
1 cup	chocolate 1% milk
1 cup	1% milk
1	string cheese (from 2% milk)
½ cup	non-fat cottage cheese
½ cup	non-fat frozen yogurt
1 cup	skim milk
1 cup	non-fat yogurt

EGGS	
¼ cup	egg substitute
4	egg whites
2	eggs
2	omega-3 eggs

LEGUMES	
½ cup	cooked or canned beans
½ cup	peas (cooked or canned)
1 cup	calcium-fortified light soymilk
½ cup	lentils (cooked)
½ cup	soymilk
1 Tbsp	almond butter
1 Tbsp	peanut butter (natural)
½ ounces	raw nuts

SUPPLEMENTS	
1 serving	protein supplement, such as EAS Myoplex Lite RTD
1 bar	protein supplement, such as EAS Myoplex Lite nutrition bar
1 packet	protein supplement, such as EAS Myoplex Lite powder

VEGETABLES	
GREEN	
1 cup	dark green leafy vegetables
½ cup	cooked/steamed vegetables
1½ cup	asparagus (cooked)
½ cup	broccoli (cooked)
1 cup	broccoli (raw)
1 cup	Brussels sprouts (cooked)
½ cup	celery (cooked)
1 cup	celery (raw)
1 cup	collard greens (cooked)
1 cup	cucumber (raw)
½ cup	green beans (cooked)
1 cup	green beans (raw)
1 cup	green veggie salad
1 cup	kale (raw)
½ cup	lettuce
1 cup	spinach (raw)
WHITE	
½ cup	cabbage (cooked)
1 cup	cabbage (raw)
½ cup	cauliflower (cooked)
1 cup	cauliflower (raw)
½ cup	onions (cooked)
1 cup	onions (raw)
½ cup	water chestnuts (cooked)
1 cup	water chestnuts (raw)
RED	
½ cup	tomatoes, beets

½ cup	salsa, tomato sauce

ORANGE

½ cup	carrots (cooked)
1 cup	carrots (raw)

MIXED COLORS

½ cup	peppers (cooked)
1 cup	peppers (raw)
½ cup	stir-fry vegetables (cooked)
1 cup	stir-fry vegetables (raw/frozen)
¾ cup	vegetable juice
½ cup	zucchini (cooked)
1 cup	zucchini (raw)

FRUITS

RED

1 small	apple
½ cup	applesauce (unsweetened)
12	cherries
1 cup	raspberries
1¼ cups	strawberries (whole)
¼ cup	watermelon (cubed)
½ med.	grapefruit

ORANGE

1 cup	cantaloupe (cubed)
1 med.	orange, nectarine, or peach
1 large	tangerine

YELLOW

½ large	banana
¾ cup	pineapple chunks (in own juice)

BLUE/PURPLE

1 cup	blackberries or boysenberries
¾ cup	blueberries
14	grapes

2 small	plums
3	prunes (dried plums)
2 Tbsp	raisins

GREEN

1 cup	honeydew (cubed)
1 small	kiwi
1 small	pear

MIXED COLORS

2 Tbsp	dried fruit
½ cup	fresh fruit salad
¾ cup	fruit juice (100% juice)
1 cup	mixed berries (fresh or frozen)

FATS: CHOOSE OFTEN

1 Tbsp	almond butter
11	almonds
¼ med.	avocado
10 large	black olives
1½ tsp	canola oil
2 Tbsp	flaxseed
1½ tsp	flaxseed oil
15 large	green olives
1½ tsp	olive oil
1 Tbsp	peanut butter (natural)
8	pecan halves
2 Tbsp	pumpkin seeds
2 Tbsp	sesame seeds
2 Tbsp	sunflower seeds
1½ tsp	corn oil
2 tsp	margarine
3 Tbsp	reduced-fat mayonnaise
3 Tbsp	reduced-fat salad dressing
1½ tsp	safflower oil

1½ tsp	soybean oil
1½ tsp	sunflower oil
7	walnut halves
3 Tbsp	guacamole
FATS: CHOOSE LESS OFTEN	
2 tsp	butter (stick)
1 Tbsp	butter (whipped)
1 ounce	cheese
1 slice	cheese
1½ tsp	coconut oil
1 Tbsp	cream cheese

¼ Tbsp	half-and-half
2 tsp	mayonnaise
2 slices	reduced-fat cheese
1½ Tbsp	reduced-fat butter
3 Tbsp	reduced-fat cream cheese
4 Tbsp	reduced-fat sour cream
3 Tbsp	sour cream
2 slices	turkey bacon
1 link	turkey sausage

Healthy Meal Components

These tables will help you create healthful meals custom-tailored to your nutritional needs. Make sure you eat your meal or snack within thirty minutes after your workout.

Now that you have an idea of how to assemble your meals, use the simple chart below. To determine which of the three zones you fall under, find your age in the left column and your weight in the top row. From there you can see what portions of grains, protein/ dairy, fruits, vegetables, and fats to assemble for each meal.

	110	120	130	140	150	160	170	180	190	200+
25	1	1	1	2	2	2	3	3	3	3
30	1	1	1	1	2	2	2	3	3	3
35	1	1	1	1	2	2	2	3	3	3
40	1	1	1	1	1	2	2	2	3	3
45	1	1	1	1	1	2	2	2	3	3
50	1	1	1	1	1	1	2	2	2	3
55	1	1	1	1	1	1	2	2	2	3
60	1	1	1	1	1	1	1	2	2	2

FUELING TIMES						
ZONE 1	**BREAKFAST**	**SNACK**	**LUNCH**	**SNACK**	**DINNER**	**SNACK**
Grains	1	**	1	1	1	**
Protein/Dairy	1	**	1	**	1	1
Fruits	1	1	1	**	**	1
Veggies	**	**	3	**	3	**
Fats	1	1	1	1	1	**
or						
Meal Replacement Bar/Shake		1		1		1

FUELING TIMES						
ZONE 2	**BREAKFAST**	**SNACK**	**LUNCH**	**SNACK**	**DINNER**	**SNACK**
Grains	1–2		1–2	1	1	
Protein/Dairy	1		1		1	1
Fruits	1	1				1
Veggies			3		3	
Fats	1	1	1	1	1	
or						
Meal Replacement Bar/Shake		1		1		1

FUELING TIMES						
ZONE 3	**BREAKFAST**	**SNACK**	**LUNCH**	**SNACK**	**DINNER**	**SNACK**
Grains	2		2	1	1–2	
Protein/Dairy	1		1		1	1
Fruits	1	1		1		1
Veggies			3		3	
Fats	1	1	1	1	1	
or						
Meal Replacement Bar/Shake		1		1		1

Core Grocery List

General Shopping Tips

Stay focused. • Go in with a plan. • Avoid products at the heads of the aisles. • Watch out at the checkout! • Explore one, new healthy food with each shopping trip.

Here's an aisle-by-aisle look at how to approach your grocery store shopping.

BAKERY

100% whole-wheat bread (look for at least 3 grams of fiber)

Pumpernickel bread/products

Sourdough bread/products

CEREAL AISLE

Bran cereal

Kashi cereal (my personal favorite), unsweetened varieties

Slow-cooked oats

CANNED FOODS

Black beans

Chickpeas

Kidney beans

Navy beans

Pinto beans

Fruit (canned in its own juice) with no sugar added

Tuna, water-packed

Chicken, water-packed

DELI SECTION

TIP: Avoid deli salads and fried foods.

Deli meats, lean and reduced-fat (turkey, chicken, roast beef, ham)

Hummus

Rotisserie chicken (remove skin and remove surface fat with a paper towel)

BAKING, SNACK, AND CONDIMENT AISLES

Almonds

Cashews

Peanuts

Sunflower seeds

Canola oil

Olive oil

High-protein meal-replacement bars

Mustard

Almond butter

Peanut butter, natural

Salad dressing, low-fat

Vinegar, balsamic or red wine (for salads)

MEAT AND SEAFOOD AISLES

Chicken, skinless, white meat

Ground beef, 96% fat-free

Red meat and pork, lean

Turkey, white meat

Salmon and other fish

DAIRY SECTION

TIP: Avoid whole-milk products.

Cheese, reduced-fat

Cottage cheese, 2%, 1%, or fat-free

String cheese

Juices, 100% juice, no sugar added

Milk, 1% or fat-free

Yogurt—natural low-fat plain with no added sugar, or plain Greek

FROZEN FOOD

Fruits

Ice cream, low-fat, low-sugar

Soy yogurt or ice cream

Juices, 100% juice, no sugar added

Kashi waffles

Vegetables

PRODUCE SECTION

TIP: Stock up! Cut and package produce to eat later.

Apples, red or green

Apricots

Avocados

Bananas

Blueberries

Broccoli

Brussels sprouts

Carrots

Cauliflower

Cucumbers

Edamame

Grapefruits

Grapes, red

Green beans

Kale

Kiwis

Oranges

Pears

Bell peppers, green, red, yellow

Romaine lettuce

Spinach

Strawberries

Sweet potatoes

Tofu

Tomatoes

PHARMACY

Calcium with vitamin D for women

Fish oil capsules

Krill oil (if preferred instead of fish oil)

Multivitamin

Whey protein powder or meal replacement powder (such as EAS Myoplex)

Rice protein

BEVERAGE AISLES

Coffee, regular and decaf

Powdered beverages (such as Crystal Light)

Juices, 100% juice, no sugar added

Tea (green, white, and black)

Water, bottled

Wine, red

SERVING SIZES

VEGETABLES: 1 cup raw leafy vegetables, ½ cup cooked or raw vegetables, ¾ cup vegetable juice, ½ cup cooked dry beans

FRUITS: 1 medium fruit (1 medium apple or 1 medium pear), ½ cup canned or chopped fruit, or ¾ cup fruit juice

BREADS AND CEREALS: 1 slice of bread, 1 cup ready-to-eat cereal, ½ cup cooked rice or pasta

PROTEIN: 3–4 ounces meat (size of a deck of cards)

FATS: 1 tablespoon olive oil, 2 tablespoons peanut butter, handful of nuts

DAIRY: 1 cup milk, ½ cup cottage cheese, 1 ounce or 1 slice of cheese

The Costco Diet?

I hail from Sequim, Washington, not far from the headquarters of Costco Wholesale, the popular warehouse shopping company that sells everything from electronics to clothes, books to wine, furniture to tires, and, of course, food.

There's a misperception about Costco and its competitors that they only sell food in bulk sizes fit for a family of twelve. Actually many items in warehouse stores are the same size you might find in grocery stores, at a fraction of the cost.

I'm a big fan of Costco, especially its commitment to customer service and providing quality merchandise at affordable prices. My coauthor Pete Williams has reached the point where he rarely shops anywhere else. Talk about keeping life simple.

Here's a look at how to simplify your nutrition planning.

Rotisserie chicken: These are an excellent value at $5.99. Remove the fatty skin and you have enough for one meal plus leftovers. If you buy two, you can carve the second one up and take care of several lunches and perhaps another dinner. Other great protein sources available at Costco include eggs and cottage cheese.

Flank steak: This is the leanest cut of beef, yet it's juicy and flavorful. Costco portions aren't small, but if you're cooking for only one or two, you can freeze half of it.

Wild salmon: It's sometimes difficult to find salmon that's not farm-raised, which contains higher levels of chlorinated compounds known as polychlorinated biphenyls (PCBs). Costco sells wild salmon, some of which is already marinated.

Vegetables: Go for the mixed dark greens available in boxes or bags. Organic spinach comes in large bags or plastic tubs with a short-term expiration date. Spinach is versatile—you can use it to anchor salads or cook it in olive oil and serve as a side dish for dinner. Asparagus and broccoli come in larger packages and can be enjoyed several times over the course of the week. At our house asparagus is considered finger food.

Berries: Berries are one of the best sources of antioxidants and they provide flavor as an oatmeal topping or part of a dessert. The price of blueberries fluctuates wildly over the course of the year, depending on whether Costco can obtain them from local farmers or must ship them from greater distances. You usually can find blackberries and strawberries as well. Frozen berries are always a good option.

Olive oil: This can be a bigger-ticket item, so it pays to buy in bulk. Costco's private-label "Kirkland" extra virgin olive oil is a good value and a rich source of healthy fats as a salad dressing or as a marinade for spinach and asparagus.

Tomatoes: Rich in antioxidants, tomatoes are a staple of any high-performance diet. Costco sells them in all sizes, from grape to full-size.

Oatmeal: There's perhaps no simpler, better breakfast than old-fashioned Quaker oatmeal. Costco sells a large double-bag box that will last two months, even if you eat oatmeal every day for breakfast. Steel-cut oats is a terrific option, as well, and can sometimes be found at Costco.

Whey protein powder: Whey is a by-product of cheese manufacturing and includes many essential amino acids that boost the immune system and promote overall good health. Protein powder, such as EAS whey protein, can be found in chocolate and vanilla powder and can be mixed with oatmeal to give your breakfast some potent protein. It's also good as part of a pre-workout shooter or mixed with berries as a smoothie.

Nuts: They're not cheap, so it pays to buy in bulk. You can put them in salads, mix them into post-workout recovery shakes, and even eat them alone as a midafternoon snack to get some healthy fats. Almonds, walnuts, and pecans are good choices. Freeze to keep fresh.

Brown rice, whole-wheat couscous, whole-wheat pasta: Since we make this category a minor portion of Core Performance nutrition, you might be better served with smaller packages from the grocery store. Then again, these products do have a long shelf life.

Water: Costco sells bottled water by the case. Grab some standard half-liter bottles, along with some 8-ouncers for kids or guests who might not need a full bottle. Of course, you can save money and the environment by refilling your own water bottle.

Wine: Did you know that nobody sells more wine in the United States than Costco? Because of that buying power, the savings is passed along to you. Costco wines come from all over the world, including Europe, South America, and Australia. Alcohol, even wine, should be kept in moderation, but there's perhaps no better place to pick up a quality bottle of wine for a reasonable price. My favorite is pinot noir, but Costco has everything to satisfy your wine palate.

With just these thirteen items, you can feed yourself for a week. It's not all you should eat, but it could account for more than 80 percent of what you consume, more than enough to keep yourself on budget and, more important, on track with the Core Performance nutrition program.

Protein: The Key to Performance

When it comes to protein, many people struggle to find the happy medium. Some people don't get enough, while others follow diets dangerously low on carbs and go overboard on protein.

Protein builds, maintains, and restores muscle. It's responsible for healthy blood cells, key enzymes, and a strong immune system. In order to build and maintain muscle, you must consume protein with enough carbohydrate calories to provide your body with energy. Otherwise your body will tap into the protein for fuel. Using protein for energy is inefficient and ineffective for performance.

Just as athletes have higher carbohydrate needs than the average person, they also need more protein. This is also true for women who incorporate strength training into their regimen, as in the Core Performance Women program.

Exercise produces a catabolic effect, breaking down precious lean body mass. By consuming adequate protein, both throughout the day and especially after training sessions, we help our bodies minimize and reverse this effect and jump-start our road to recovery.

As a general rule of thumb, you need to consume between 0.6 and 0.8 gram of protein per pound of body weight. If you weigh, say, 140 pounds, you want to shoot for between 84 and 112 grams of protein per day. Generally speaking, the leaner and more active you are, the higher your protein intake should be. (See chart on page 90.)

That might sound like a lot of protein—and it is a significant amount—but consider how much protein is in these common foods:

Chicken (4 ounces, skinless, the size of a deck of cards): 35 grams

Cod or salmon (6 ounces): 40 grams

Tuna (6 ounces, packed in water): 40 grams

Lean pork (4 ounces): 35 grams

Lean red meat (4 ounces): 35 grams

Tofu (6 ounces): 30 grams

Cottage cheese (1 cup, 1% or 2% fat): 28 grams

Milk (1 cup of 1%, 2%, or fat-free): 8 grams

1 egg: 6 grams

1 egg white: 3 grams

Protein intake should be split up over the course of the day, and it should be included in every meal. Protein helps to stabilize energy, promotes satiety, and also revs up the metabolism. Your body has to work a little harder to digest protein; therefore your metabolism gets a bit of a jolt each time you include it in a meal. By including a protein source with each of your meals and your post-workout recovery shake, you will easily and effectively satisfy your protein needs.

Here's a good rule of thumb about protein: "The fewer legs, the better." The fewer legs something had when it was alive, the better its ratio of protein to healthy fat.

Fish, for instance, is a healthy source of protein, assuming that it's not fried. Fish such as salmon and albacore tuna also provide an optimal ratio of omega-3 and omega-6 fatty acids. The omega-3 fatty acids help to promote cardiovascular health and decrease inflammation. Other great sources of protein from seafood include mussels, scallops, and several fish with lots of legs: shrimp and lobster. Chicken is also a wonderful source of protein, provided the skin is removed and the meat is not fried.

Meat from four-legged creatures can be good provided it's a lean cut. Lean red meat is a source of important nutrients such as iron, zinc, and B vitamins. Grass-fed red meat products are preferable than corn-fed options since those animals typically had less exposure to hormones and pesticides. Even the fattier cuts of grass-fed beef have a better fatty-acid profile, providing omega-3 fatty acids. Lean cuts of pork and ham also are good sources of protein.

Dairy products provide protein, calcium, and vitamin D for strong bones. When you

Daily Protein Intake

WEIGHT (LB)	PROTEIN NEEDED (G)
90	54–72
100	60–80
110	66–99
120	72–96
130	78–104
140	84–112
150	90–120
160	96–128
170	102–136
180	108–144

start to consider how much protein you really need to eat, you may think that it sounds like a lot, but in reality it's a manageable amount.

Eggs are a tremendous source of protein. In the last decade eggs have been cast as something of a dietary villain, linked to heart disease and high cholesterol. Instead let's focus on the benefits of eggs. They are a great source of choline, a dietary nutrient essential for normal cell function and brain health. Eggs also are a source of lutein and zeaxanthin, two carotenoids that promote eye health. Eggs also provide protein and healthy fats with minimal calories. The whole egg will keep you feeling fuller longer and provide you with more nutrients than just eating egg whites. So go ahead and eat the whole egg.

You should also incorporate a post-workout recovery shake mix into your routine. That mix will contain 10 to 25 grams of protein per serving, along with carbs. If you have one or two shakes a day, along with some combination of poultry and fish for lunch and dinner and a breakfast that includes yogurt or eggs, you'll easily meet your daily protein goal.

Fabulous Fat

Contrary to popular belief, fat will not make you fat. Unfortunately, thanks to the aggressive anti-fat marketing campaigns of the 1980s, most people believe that if you eat fat, you become fat.

There's some truth to that, of course. Not all fat is good, and too much of anything will contribute to additional body fat. But fats are crucial to good health and the makeup of cell membranes. Fats are needed for the absorption of certain vitamins and antioxidants: vitamin A (immune function and wound healing), vitamin D (bone health and general well-being), vitamin E (involved with the workings of vitamins A and C and helps to protect the cells), and vitamin K (normal blood clotting function). Fats release energy slowly, keeping the body satiated and regulating blood sugar, thus lowering glycemic response to other foods. Research also confirms that fats send signals to the brain that then make us feel full. Good fats provide powerful nutrients for cellular repair of the joints, organs, skin, and hair. Special fatty acids, specifically omega-3s (EPA and DHA), found in fatty fish, fish oil, walnuts, flaxseeds, and flaxseed oil, also help with cognitive ability, mental clarity, mood, PMS, and memory retention, and they have strong anti-inflammatory properties. These essential fats are often overlooked. The fact that their name incorporates the word *essential* means that they must come from the diet. I cannot stress too much the importance of incorporating these fats into your diet on a daily basis or choosing a fish oil or omega-3 supplement to complement your diet.

Take pains to avoid saturated fats, which are usually found in meat and dairy foods and are solid at room temperature. Saturated fats raise serum cholesterol, clog arteries, and pose a risk to the heart.

We also want to stay away from trans fats, which raise bad (LDL) cholesterol but do not raise good (HDL) cholesterol. Artery-clogging trans fats are found in processed foods such as cookies, crackers, pies, pastries, and margarine. They're also found in

Supplements for Women

Even a strong nutrition program like Core Performance Women isn't always enough to give your body what it needs to fortify itself against the stresses of everyday life. Here are some supplements you might want to consider:

- A multivitamin that offers a full spectrum of antioxidants and B vitamins and can fill in the gaps of your nutrition plan, sending in reinforcements in the fight against cellular-damaging free radicals, keeping our bodies and minds healthy.
- Calcium and vitamin D, both found in milk, work together to prevent several chronic diseases. They keep bones and teeth strong and also help with blood clotting, nerve function, muscle contraction and relaxation, and enzyme regulation. You can't go wrong adding a calcium/vitamin D supplement to your nutrition program.
- Fish oil provides powerful omega-3 fatty acids, which have anti-inflammatory properties and are essential for good cardiovascular health and mental clarity. Everyone should have a bottle of fish oil or fish oil capsules in their pantry. If fish oil gives you a case of the burps, krill oil is a good substitute.

fried foods and in smaller amounts in meat and some dairy products. Thankfully, food manufacturers must now list trans fat amounts on their product labels.

However, even if the label says "no trans fat," there is a chance that there may be some trans fat in the product. If there is less than 0.5 gram of trans fat per serving, the FDA allows the manufacturer to label it as containing "no trans fats." Yep—the FDA allows the manufacturer to round down. So read the label *and* the ingredients list. If the words "hydrogenated" or "fractionated" appear in any of the first four ingredients, the product likely contains trans fats. If you are choosing minimally processed whole foods, you should not have to worry about trans fats.

The best fats come out of nuts, seeds, and fish oils. Nuts and seeds are a con-

Clean Eating, Clean House

Can eating cleaner make your *house* cleaner? Yes, if you follow this rule: The Fewer Crumbs the Better.

Everything that produces crumbs—cookies, crackers, chips, snack foods, doughnuts, bread, and nearly all cereals—has no place in the Core Performance Women nutrition program. With the exception of high-fiber, 100 percent whole-wheat products, forget about anything that produces crumbs.

So not only will you experience the physical benefits of eating better, you'll have a cleaner house as well!

venient source of protein and fiber, and they stick with you longer than many other snacks, helping to control blood sugar and appetite. Nuts are a convenient snack—a handful every day can lower your risk of heart ailments and Alzheimer's disease and can even lower cholesterol. Nuts and seeds are unsaturated fats, which do not raise cholesterol levels. The best unsaturated fats, liquid at room temperature, are found in olive oil, canola oil, Enova brand oil, and fish oils. Walnuts in particular have been linked with decreasing cholesterol and are also a good source of omega-3 fatty acids.

Fish oils also provide powerful omega-3 fatty acids, which have anti-inflammatory properties and are essential for good cardiovascular health and mental clarity. Our bodies need an optimal ratio of omega-6 to omega-3 fatty acids, generally between 4 to 1 and 10 to 1. Most diets, though, are typically much higher in omega-6 than omega-3. The omega-3 fatty acids found in salmon, mackerel, lake trout, herring, sardines, tuna, and some types of white fish cannot be made by your body, so they must come from your diet. Unless you eat fish at least three times a week, you're not getting enough omega-3s.

Everyone should have a bottle of fish oil or fish oil capsules in their pantry. Fish oil is high in omega-3 and some omega-6 fatty acids. The two components to look at on your fish oil supplement are EPA and DHA. It is recommended that you get a total of 1 to 3 grams of combined EPA and DHA per day, not just 1 to 3 grams of total fish oil. It also is recommended that you get about 500 mg of DHA for healthy brain and mood functioning. If you are pregnant and nursing, you will find DHA in the prenatal vitamins recommended by your doctor. These serve as brain food for the developing baby and also for you, so be sure to incorporate them into your daily routine. As with any supplement, check with your physician before taking the product.

Rule #2: Eat Early, Often, and Balanced

If you're a child of the 1970s or 80s like I am, you probably remember that advice Mom gave about eating "three square meals a day" and avoiding between-meal snacks. It probably was intended for people who were eating only one or two decent meals a day. Today, however, we know that if you want to control your blood sugar level and energy level to improve concentration, regulate your appetite, and build lean body mass, you must eat *six* small- to medium-size meals or snacks a day. That means you need to eat, on average, every three hours. Think of yourself as "grazing" throughout the day instead of sitting for three big meals. If you can't control your blood sugar levels, you're going to have wild fluctuations in energy levels and moods and an impaired ability to concentrate.

Remember this formula: "3 for 3." Eat all three nutrients (protein, carbohydrate, fat) every three hours for optimal energy and body composition.

Like a fire, your metabolism is in constant need of fuel. If you let it go for a long time without adding logs, the fire smolders and dies. Each time you eat (or add fuel) to the fire, it cranks up your metabolism and burns more calories to digest the food. You have an efficient metabolism.

By following the Core Performance Women program, you'll create this constantly burning fire. If you don't continually fuel the fire, you're going to draw from your valuable lean muscle mass and smolder. If you don't eat often, the most readily available substance for the body to consume is muscle—not fat, as is commonly believed. The body is actually remarkably resistant to fat loss and will turn to lean muscle mass first, keeping that stored fat in reserve as long as possible.

Many women try to stay thin by not eating. They deprive their bodies of nutrients and, while they might look healthy, their bodies may be really out of balance. When your body is not properly nourished, it travels a slippery slope of hormonal imbalance, decreased energy, inability to recover efficiently, and compromised lean muscle mass.

The last thing you want to do is lose the lean mass you've worked so hard to achieve. After all, the more lean mass you have, the more calories you burn at rest. Plus, less lean mass puts your body at a greater risk for injury. Lean mass produces power, stabilizes joints, promotes movement, and is critical for optimal performance.

By eating six "meals," we're going to graze throughout the day. But these are going to be healthy meals. Women, perhaps more so than men, have a tendency toward mindless eating, consuming food when they don't necessarily realize it. A very funny man named Rob Becker created a one-man play called *Defending the Caveman* in which he explained that men and women have been wired differently since the days of the cavemen. The main difference between the sexes, he suggests, is that men are hunters and women are gatherers. Men remain focused on one pursuit, to the exclusion of all else. Women take their time, not wanting to miss anything. Shopping is how Becker most effectively argues this point.

Becker also suggests that women traditionally gathered as much food as they could to feed the entire tribe and to put some away for the winter. There's nothing wrong with that, but what we don't want to do is consume food just because it's available.

Our six meals need not be long, sit-down affairs. (We eat to live, not live to eat, right?) Three of them could be a little larger and a traditional combination of energy-rich, clean foods. One could be a post-workout recovery shake, another a piece of fruit with nuts and a piece of string cheese or a meal replacement bar. Many of these options can fit in your purse, desk drawer, or diaper bag.

I'm not a big fan of the word *snack*, since it's come to refer to junk food or something you might feed your dog. We do, however, want to have three smaller snacks or "mini-meals" to go with our three moderate-size meals, what we think of as breakfast, lunch, and dinner. Or you could have six meals of equal size. Just remember to make sure that you account for all three nutrients (carbs, protein, and fat) every three hours. You should strive for a balance between carbs, proteins, and good fats in each of your meals.

These meals should start early—as soon as you get up. One nutrition cliché that is in fact true is that breakfast is the most important meal of the day. Your body has been fasting since you went to bed, so it's important that you "break the fast" not long after rising and keep your body fueled all day long. I can't think of an easier, healthier breakfast than a cup of old-fashioned oatmeal and skim milk or yogurt.

Many women insist they're not hungry for breakfast, consuming nothing but coffee on the go. If this is you, let's examine this mindset. Why are you not hungry in the morning? Do you eat too much at night? It's possible to get into a pattern that makes eating breakfast a challenge. If you skip breakfast and push on until lunch, you're probably going to be famished. Not surprisingly, you overeat for lunch. As a result, you're not that hungry for dinner but eat a large portion anyway, since, after all, it's dinner. Women who are not hungry for breakfast tend to have issues with reactive eating (responding to hunger and environment) and portion control (eating too much because of hunger). Just beginning your day with breakfast will place you on the right path toward fueling yourself more efficiently and proactively, which will create a better you, inside and out.

I'd rather you eat *anything* for breakfast than skip the meal. When I coached college athletes, I had such difficulty getting them to eat breakfast that I all but begged

Five Simple Breakfasts to Keep You Going:

- A slice of whole-wheat toast with 1 tablespoon peanut butter; low-fat yogurt mixed with 1 cup of berries
- One cup of unsweetened Kashi cereal, half a banana, ¼ cup walnuts, and 1 cup skim milk
- 1 whole-wheat English muffin, 1 cooked egg, 1 slice low-fat cheese, and 1 cup strawberries
- ½ cup slow-cooked oats with ¼ cup pecans, ¼ cup raisins, and 2 hard-boiled eggs
- 1 whole-wheat tortilla rolled up with 3 ounces turkey and 1 tablespoon low-fat cream cheese, along with an apple

them to eat leftover pizza instead of going hungry. That's how important breakfast is, especially if you work out early in the morning—you need to fuel up before training. Research suggests that those who eat before training sessions or even a challenging day at the office can go harder and longer.

As you build your meals through the rest of your day, remember the three nutrients and judge your meals with your visual cues. With a little practice, all you will have to do is look at the plate and you'll know whether it will serve your needs. Typically your plate should consist mostly of colorful vegetables. There should be a piece of meat the size of a deck of cards and a fist-size portion of brown rice or whole-wheat pasta. There also should be some good fat in the form of something like nuts and healthy oils.

I recommend that you "eat a rainbow often," which not only refers to the bright colors of fiber-rich fruits and vegetables that should be part of every meal but also reminds you to eat six small meals and snacks daily.

The Mini-Meal

So what are some good mini-meals? Meal replacement bars and ready-to-drink shakes that contain whey protein powder, such as those produced by EAS, are handy snacks when you're in a rush. Try not to rely on them, however, since natural foods offer valuable nutrients your body needs. By stocking your purse, desk drawer, or diaper bag with natural foods, you'll snack great throughout the day. By snacking on a combination of carbohydrates, healthy fats, and lean protein every two to three hours, you'll spike your metabolism, boost energy, and feel fuller longer.

Use the foods below to create the snacks of your choice in three simple steps. (Single serving size noted in parentheses.)

STEP 1—Choose one minimally processed carbohydrate for energy.

Packets of Kashi oatmeal (1 packet)

100 percent whole-wheat bread (1 to 2 slices)

Whole-wheat crackers (5 to 10; check the serving size)

High-fiber cereal (½ to 1 cup)

Seasonal fruits and veggies (bite-size—1 to 2 cups—lots of volume, minimal calories)

STEP 2—Pair with one lean protein to rev your metabolism.

Beef or turkey jerky (1 ounce—4 or 5 pieces)

Rule #3: Hydrate

What if I told you there was something you could drink that would increase your energy levels, improve the quality of your skin, keep your muscles and joints lubricated, improve your overall health, make you look younger, and prevent you from overeating? What if I also told you that this drink is readily available for little to no cost and you could drink as much of it as you wanted?

Canned tuna or chicken (3-ounce can)

Low-fat yogurt or string cheese (if you have a mini fridge to store it—1 cup low-fat)

Low-fat cottage cheese (if you have a mini fridge to store it—½ to 1 cup)

Lean deli meat (if you have a mini fridge to store it—3 to 4 ounces)

STEP 3—Add a healthy fat to increase satiety.

Raw almonds, pecans, and walnuts (1 ounce, ¼ cup, or the amount in 1 small handful—to fit in the palm of your hand)

Natural peanut butter or almond butter (1 to 2 teaspoons)

Hummus (¼ cup)

Low-fat cheese (½ to 1 slice)

STEP 4—Mix and match the foods above as you wish or try these six easy snacks.

1. Yogurt with a ¼ cup high-fiber cereal, 2 tablespoons raw nuts, and ½ cup berries

2. Peanut butter and banana—or make it a sandwich

3. Apple, string cheese, and a handful of almonds

4. Baby carrots dipped in hummus with side of beef jerky

5. Kashi oatmeal, 1 tablespoon natural peanut butter, or a handful of pecans

6. 1 hard-boiled egg

My guess is you'd rush to stock up on this revolutionary liquid. Actually, you already have an unlimited supply in your home of this perfect beverage we often take for granted.

Indeed, for all of the advances in technology, we still have not come up with something better than water. Unfortunately, though, we tend to replace it with inferior beverages ranging from soda to coffee to alcohol.

Stay Thin—Eat Breakfast!

Don't just take my word for it. In a study by the Breakfast Research Institute published in the *American Journal of Clinical Nutrition* late in 2008, researchers supported the theory that breakfast eaters are less likely to be overweight. Eating a high-quality breakfast, they stress, is the key.

Research has long suggested that people who eat a bowl of cereal for breakfast weigh less than either those who skip breakfast or those who scarf down eggs with sausage or bacon.

What makes the latest study so intriguing is the difference in findings between men and women. Men who ate a healthy breakfast generally weighed less than those who ate poorly or not at all. Among women, breakfast eaters—regardless of what they ate—tended to weigh less than those who skipped the meal.

This supports my "cold pizza" prescription, but I'd still rather women eat a healthy breakfast. The study recommends choosing breakfast foods low in "energy density," low in calories for a given amount of food. Though this seems like awkward phrasing—don't we want high energy density?—it makes sense. Foods like fruit, vegetables, and high-fiber whole grains are low in calories given the amount of food. You'll stay satiated longer and feel energized longer.

Confectionery products like Danish pastries and doughnuts have a high energy density, which is to say lots of calories for the amount of food. They'll give you a quick sugar rush, but you'll crash and be hungry again soon.

Bottom line: Any breakfast is better than no breakfast, but a healthier a.m. meal is best.

By drinking the proper amount of water every day, you could accomplish 25 percent more. Just drink enough water before, during, and after exercise. Try to drink ½ to 1 ounce of water per pound of body weight per day. Or just divide your body weight by two. Drink 2 cups of water first thing in the morning. Invest in a one-liter stainless-steel water bottle. Take it to work or as you run errands and try to fill it three times over the course of the day.

Proper hydration regulates appetite. Often when people think they're hungry they're really just thirsty. Staying hydrated throughout the day will help you keep the weight off. Get in touch with your hunger by asking yourself if you are truly hungry or just thirsty.

When it comes to drinking—not just alcohol, but all drinking—the number-one rule to remember is this: Don't drink calories. It's the single easiest way to get a handle on your nutrition program. If you replace soft drinks, juices, sports drinks, and alcohol with water or natural teas, you'll cut down on calories and sugar. (But stay clear of "specialty waters," which are marketed for their vitamins, but many are packed full of sugar and calories. Check the labels on everything you drink!) Always keep your bottle of water close at hand; that way you're more likely to grab water instead of sugary drinks.

Water can retard the aging process. Because of dehydration, inactivity, and trauma from daily life, the connective tissues around our muscles and joints dry up over time, like chew toys for dogs that start out soft and pliable and end up stiff and brittle. Drinking lots of water prevents this process while improving your muscle tissue and flexibility.

As discussed in the last chapter, caffeine should not be used as a daily energy source. Following the Core Performance Women workout and nutrition program means you won't need to rely on stimulants just to get through the day.

Black coffee or espresso that isn't loaded with cream and sugar has antioxidant properties, and when consumed in moderation can help meet your antioxidant needs and, of course, increase alertness. However, you should also derive antioxidants from a variety of fruits and vegetables and from other drinks such as green, white, or black tea, each of which has different protective antioxidant properties.

Soda is loaded with sugar and fat-producing high-fructose corn syrup. Did you know there are roughly fifteen spoonfuls of sugar in just one 12-ounce can of soda?

Diet sodas are no substitute for water either. Even though they have fewer calories than their fully loaded counterparts, they still deliver artificial flavors, colors, sweeteners, and chemicals to your body. Diet soda typically contains about six packets of Splenda per 12-ounce can. That's a lot of artificial sweetener, especially if you consume multiple sodas a day. There's nothing wrong with an *occasional* diet soda, but it should not be a habitual source of hydration. Instead just reach for clean drinks: water and naturally calorie-free teas.

Don't assume that sports drinks are an adequate substitute for water, either. If you're training in extreme heat, sports drinks can be critical for performance. But they were not meant to be consumed throughout the day while sitting at your desk or watching television. Many are loaded with fast-digesting carbohydrates that spike blood sugar and ultimately contribute to body fat if not needed to fuel activity. Don't get me wrong; I'm a fan of sports drinks. But only when they're used to replace electrolytes and improve performance in intense activity in the heat lasting sixty minutes or more.

Alcohol not only is loaded with calories (7 empty calories per gram), but it wreaks havoc with sleep. Women tend to favor sweeter, more colorful drinks, and these are loaded with sugar. Some heavy drinkers try to lose weight by drinking straight alcohol. After all, it reduces calories! I would not recommend this for any number of health and safety reasons. Bottom line: A high-performance lifestyle keeps alcohol in moderation. Ideally you will limit alcohol intake to an occasional glass of red wine, which, according to several studies, reduces the risk of cardiovascular disease and Alzheimer's disease.

REMEMBER: A shot of gin or whiskey contains 50 calories and a shot of rum or Southern Comfort has 80. When you add the calories from mixers, it's easy to see how an average of one or two nights of hard drinking can pack on the pounds quickly.

I know it's tough to change drinking habits, since they are such an ingrained part of daily life. But there's no easier way to maintain consistent energy levels, regulate appetite, boost performance in sports, and improve overall health than to substitute water for whatever kind of soda, caffeinated beverage, or alcoholic drink dominates your life.

Drinking Calories

It's easy to see how consuming just a few alcoholic beverages can account for a significant number of calories.

BRAND	CALORIES
Budweiser	145
Coors Light	102
Miller Genuine Draft	143
Michelob	155
Sierra Nevada Pale Ale	200
Samuel Adams Boston Lager	160
Heineken	150
Corona	148
Guinness Extra Stout	153
TYPE	**CALORIES**
Cabernet Sauvignon (red)	90
Merlot (red)	95
Chianti (red)	100
Chardonnay (white)	90
Sauvignon Blanc (white)	80
Port (Ruby)	185
TYPE	**CALORIES**
Gin and Tonic	200
Vodka Cranberry	220
Bloody Mary	180
Margarita	Up to 500
Long Island Iced Tea	Up to 550

My coauthor, Pete Williams, used to drink five or six diet sodas a day. He'd put away even more on days when he ate out, not realizing how often the server refilled his glass. Now he follows what he calls the "Bible Beverage Plan," drinking nothing but water, including water mixed with post-workout recovery mixes, and an occasional

Step off the Scale

Should you expect to gain weight or lose weight with this program?

That depends. If you step on a scale, it just gives you a number. It doesn't tell you how much muscle or lean mass you have. I can find two people the same height and weight that look dramatically different because of their body compositions. One might wear a size 8, the other a size 4. That's because a pound of fat takes up far more space than a pound of lean mass.

People tend to lose lean mass and gain fat as they age, almost a pound per year after the age of twenty-five. That's why a woman who weighs the same in her mid-forties as she did in her mid-twenties can look much different. If she has not been training and following a proper nutrition program, she's no doubt moved up a few sizes.

We want to be less concerned with weight and more concerned with our ratio of lean mass to fat. With this program you should expect to gain lean mass and lose fat. Remember, though, that a pound of lean mass takes up far less space than a pound of fat. If you're someone in reasonably good shape when you start this program, you could gain weight and look far leaner—or, as some might say, "skinnier"—losing inches off your waistline.

I had the good fortune for several years to train Mia Hamm, one of the best soccer players of all time, male or female. Mia told me that by the end of her career she weighed ten pounds more than she did in college. But she was leaner and stronger.

Mia never wanted to reveal her weight. She wasn't ashamed of it; she just didn't want young women to use that weight as a benchmark, since everyone is different. The idea is to create the optimum ratio of lean mass and fat for your high-performance lifestyle. How will that translate on the scale?

It all depends on your height, frame, and genetics. But regardless of those variables, the idea is to maintain lean mass and lose fat.

If you're someone who begins this program overweight, you might not lose as much "scale weight" as you expect. But since you're reducing fat and increasing muscle, you'll look leaner and end up stronger than with traditional diet plans that promote weight loss, which is usually temporary.

glass of wine. He feels better, gets more benefit from his workouts, has healthier teeth, and no longer relies on caffeine to get through the day. And he saves money to boot.

Pete eats plenty of fruit, so he's getting the benefits of juice—plus all of the fiber and other nutrients that would have been squeezed out during juicing. He proves that you don't need anything other than what's been available since the beginning of time to stay properly hydrated.

Rule #4: Eat to Recover

Most people think of recovery and eating in terms of Thanksgiving dinner, falling asleep on the couch in a food coma by halftime of the second football game.

Rather than recovering from eating, we want to think in terms of eating to recover. This pertains not only to our post-workout recovery fueling (more on that in a moment) but also how we use food to kick-start our day-to-day recovery from the stresses of life.

I spend a lot of time in New York, and while I love the energy I feel just walking the streets of Manhattan between appointments, there's a lot of damage being inflicted on my body. There's the stress of the day, the pollutants from the streets, and the sun beating down on me. That, along with the stress of flying cross-country and dealing with a long cab ride into the city, produces a lot of damage on the cellular level that needs to be repaired. The quickest and most efficient way to do that is through some nutrient-dense foods high in fiber and antioxidants. Otherwise your immune system will be compromised.

The immune system is the foundation for overall health. By boosting the immune system, you prevent inflammation and premature aging and increase your energy levels. Not only that, it seems like there's a radiance flowing from you. People view you as more active and energetic. Your hair and skin seem healthier and more vibrant. In many respects beauty is nothing more than an expression of energy or cellular vitality.

Think about that for a moment. Even the most genetically blessed "beautiful" women will not look attractive with a battered immune system. If they're lacking energy, appearing tired and run-down from a poor nutrition program (along with perhaps too much alcohol, smoking, and too little sleep), they rob themselves of their natural beauty. They appear older than they really are. The pages of *Us Weekly* and *People* magazine are packed with candid photos of female celebrities who endure these lifestyles, sacrificing their natural beauty in large part because of what they eat and what they don't. They might look like a million bucks on television and in magazines, thanks to makeup artists, stylists, favorable lighting, and Photoshop, but in real life they're a mess.

Now let's take a woman who might be lacking in what the mass media and the fashion industry have defined as traditional beauty. She does not have access to the latest clothes and high-end stylists, but her nutrition program has given her this inner beauty that radiates outward. Her hair and skin seem to glow and she glides through life with boundless energy. She looks younger than she is and, by any measuring stick, is beautiful.

Metamucil recently staged a marketing campaign about how beauty starts from the inside. This has nothing to do with regularity or those age-old quips men make about "Well, she's got a great personality." Instead, if you recognize how everything you put in your body affects your insides and permeates to the outside, you'll be far more motivated to eat properly, for energy and recovery. By eating foods that create this beauty inside (and thus outside), you'll have a relationship with food that's healthy and create an energy and confidence that a lot of women just don't have. It's the same inside-out, centered-self philosophy we discussed earlier.

Eating to recover also refers to post-workout recovery. One of my biggest challenges with nutrition, aside from getting people to eat breakfast, is getting them to eat and refuel their bodies immediately following a workout. This is especially true with women, many of whom remain obsessed with the formula of calories-in, calories-out. They figure if they just burned 500 or however many calories working out, the last thing they want to do is put those calories right back in the tank.

This is perhaps the biggest misconception about high-performance training. One of our top goals is to create more lean mass. That in turn will burn *more* calories, both at rest and during training. If we don't eat immediately following a workout, our bodies will first turn to our hard-earned lean mass for energy. As much as we'd like to think it would turn to our fat stores, the body doesn't work that way. By losing lean mass, you're creating a body that burns calories *less* efficiently. Is that what you want? I didn't think so.

Not only that, training punishes our bodies at the cellular level. When you've finished a workout, your cells are wide open and screaming for nutrients. The quickest and easiest way to replenish them is with a post-workout recovery shake, made with a protein powder (or supplement) such as EAS Myoplex or Myoplex Lite. Prepackaged, convenient shake mixes contain an effective ratio of proteins, carbohydrates, and fat and are loaded with fiber, vitamins, and minerals. Since the shakes can be made by mixing water with a scoop or packet of powder in a covered plastic container or blender, they make a quick, easy, and portable meal that won't spoil.

The active ingredient in these shakes is whey protein. A by-product of cheese manufacturing, whey (pronounced "way") includes many essential amino acids that boost the immune system and promote overall good health.

By having a shake right after your workout, you expedite the recovery process and maximize lean muscle growth. Protein powder shakes have been a longtime component of my Athletes' Performance training centers, and the elite-level athletes

The Healing Process

Eating to recover also refers to healing from wounds and surgical incisions. A proper nutrition program will expedite the healing process, while a poor one could delay healing, leaving you with greater risk of infection and scar formation. Foods rich in vitamins A and C and zinc are especially beneficial when recovering from wounds and surgeries.

who train with us have long benefited from these products. If you go through the effort to train and move your body and don't take measures to repair it, you've wasted your workout. In fact, you've done damage to your body by breaking it down without taking measures to repair it. Whichever product you choose, look for something that's going to provide 10 to 25 grams of protein and 30 to 75 grams of carbohydrate.

Compared to your training session, post-workout nutrition is the easy part. If you don't want to consume a shake, that's fine. Depending on when you work out, just move your regularly scheduled meal or snack to within thirty minutes of your workout. You could even go for some great-tasting chocolate 1% milk. A 16-ounce glass immediately after your workout will jump-start your recovery and keep you on track until your next scheduled mini-meal. If you're someone who trains during lunch hour or before dinner, that's easy enough. Just make sure you get something with a combination of carbohydrates and protein in your system within thirty minutes of training. It will improve your energy, speed your recovery, and keep you feeling great while training day in and day out.

ONE CAVEAT: You never want your body to be deprived of key nutrients, especially when you work out. Yet many people train first thing in the morning on an empty stomach. Don't get me wrong; training is a great way to start the day. In fact, that's my only time to work out. But eat something before your workout, even if it's

Recovering from a Bender

So you've decided to throw caution to the wind, eat and drink whatever you want, and then deal with the food and beverage hangover the next day. Everyone needs such days or nights. The key is to prepare accordingly.

Before attending the feast or party, plot your meals for the rest of the week and make sure your refrigerator and pantry are stocked with healthy food. Attend the celebration and do not worry about calories, fat, or the (lack of) nutritional value of the food. Enjoy every bite; instead of inhaling it, take the time to actually taste and chew your food. This way you'll be less likely to go overboard. Either way, here's how to recover the following day:

- Do not feel guilty for your indulgences.
- Start your day off with water, green tea, a multivitamin, fish oil, and a great breakfast.
- Get in a workout. Any workout, but preferably a Core Performance session.
- Jump right back into your schedule of eating five to six clean meals a day.
- Go to bed by ten p.m. and sleep for at least eight hours.
- By the following morning you should be back to your regular high-performance program.

The important thing to remember is not to let this one-day bender derail your good habits. After all, that one off day represents just 0.27 percent of the entire year. What matters most is how you eat the following day. By employing these simple strategies, you'll avoid a tailspin of poor nutrition and jolt your metabolism to start burning strong again.

just half an apple with a handful of nuts, a slice of whole-wheat toast with natural peanut butter, yogurt, or a pre-workout "shooter" consisting of a glass of watered-down orange juice with a scoop of whey protein or simply a glass of water with the scoop of whey.

CHAPTER 6 SUMMARY: Core Performance Women nutrition consists of four simple rules. "Eating clean" refers to eating a proper balance of proteins, minimally processed carbohydrates, and good fats. By eating early (breakfast) and often, you jump-start your metabolism and keep it burning hot all day, making the body a lean, fat-burning machine. By hydrating properly, with plenty of water, it's possible to get as much as a 25 percent boost in energy while avoiding the calories that come from soda, alcohol, sports drinks, and fruit juices. Nutrition also is the key to recovery, from workouts to wounds to the stresses of life.

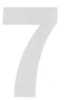

EATING ON THE GO

The biggest challenge of following any nutrition plan is implementing it on the run. It's (relatively) easy to eat right when you've purged your pantry and refrigerator at home and stocked each with quality energy sources. The trick is to prepare the same way when you're at work, running errands, or traveling.

The mindset should not change. After all, you're no doubt accustomed to planning and packing for a trip, whether for business or pleasure. If you're making a business presentation, you bring everything you need. If you're a mother with small children, you don't dare go anywhere without a backpack or diaper bag stocked with snacks and drinks.

And yet many women leave their own nutrition up in the air. If you're traveling or out running errands, chances are you're in a hurry. You lose track of time and the next thing you know, you're driving through a fast-food lane or hustling into a convenience store in search of quick nourishment.

Not only does this wreak havoc on your body but it's also time-consuming, expensive, and frustrating. You don't want to have to pay for the right to eat bad food, and waste time doing it. Plan ahead and save time and money while fueling your body for maximum energy.

Traveling presents another challenge. In recent years airlines have eliminated meal service, which is a good thing because it keeps us from eating highly processed airline food and forces us to be proactive about meal planning. Instead of buying expensive pizza and junk food in the concourse, bring a meal from home. (The bottled water you now must purchase beyond security checkpoints is expensive enough! To avoid that expense, bring an empty water bottle and fill it on the other side of security.)

On long car trips fill a cooler with bottled water, fresh fruit, vegetables, lean protein sources, healthy snack bars, and low-fat, low-sugar yogurt. Graze in the car and stop at rest areas instead of pulling off the highway and frequenting fast-food joints. Again, you'll save time and money in addition to eating right.

For longer trips, whether by car or plane, be sure to the take a meal-replacement powder to mix into a shake. If you're traveling, instead of lugging around a blender a far better choice is to use the specifically designed Core Nutrition Shake Bottle, which gives you a rotator cuff workout in the process! (They're available for less than $10 at many health food stores and at www.coreperformance.com.)

Eating in sit-down restaurants need not be challenging. It's almost always possible to order grilled chicken or fish with vegetables and a salad. Skip the bread and creamy appetizers. If a menu item isn't quite right, you usually have the option of substituting or asking for it to be prepared differently.

The key is to control your on-the-go environment as much as possible. Plan ahead.

Your Travel Checklist

These simple, compact items will save you time and money when you're on the go while keeping your body fueled properly. Pack zip-lock bags of homemade trail mix consisting of nuts, seeds, Kashi cereal, and fruit.

____ 1. Shaker bottle

____ 2. Protein powder (or supplement) packets, such as EAS Myoplex

____ 3. Green tea bags/packets

____ 4. Clif Bars

____ 5. Kashi cereal

____ 6. Nuts and seeds (raw, not honey-roasted or cocktail)

____ 7. Peanut butter (natural)

____ 8. Fruit

____ 9. Beef jerky

Bring all of the equipment you need; it need not weigh you down. Let those other travelers stand in line at the airport for a greasy six-dollar slice of pizza. Let others waste their time, money, and health at a fast-food restaurant.

On the road it's more difficult to eat right. You're generally at the mercy of restaurant menus, and you're usually pressed for time. Ideally you can find a restaurant that serves healthful food, but there will be times when you're at the mercy of a fast-food joint.

Even in these situations, don't forget your goals: peak performance and optimal health. Fast-food restaurants can be a roadblock to your nutrition goals, but with a little planning and some specific requests, you can make any fast-food restaurant meal healthier. Just remember these specific "road rules," courtesy of Amanda Carlson:

1. Take control of your food choices. Don't succumb to the mindset of "I'll get back on track when I get home."
2. Order with your mind in charge, not your stomach. This is easier to do if you do not allow yourself to get hungry.
3. Don't skip meals. You must eat every three hours.
4. Take energy bars such as Clif Bars and packets of protein powder shakes, such as EAS shakes. These are great for snacks as well as pre- and post-workout nutrition.
5. Choose a lean protein with every meal. Grilled chicken and fish, fillet of beef, and grilled pork are excellent choices.
6. Eat fruits and vegetables at every meal.
7. Drink water constantly, especially when traveling to higher altitudes.

Think about what you have already eaten throughout the day. Make choices that are low in fat and with the correct amount of carbohydrate based on your body composition goals. Remember that carbohydrates equal fuel, so if it is earlier in the day or after a workout, you may need more carbohydrate. If it is later in the day and less activity is planned, then a reduced amount of carbohydrate is needed. If you need less carbohydrate at the moment, consider the following tips:

Remove the bun from your burger or chicken sandwich, or just take off the top and eat it open-faced.
Order an extra chicken breast for your salad and skip the bread.
Leave the croutons off your salad.

Here's how to make a better choice even when there are few good options—this list notes the best options offered.

WENDY'S

- Wendy's Garden Sensation Salads with a low-fat dressing
- Grilled chicken sandwich and a side salad with a low-fat dressing
- Large chili and a side salad with a low-fat dressing
- Small chili and a baked potato with steamed broccoli
- Single cheeseburger with no mayo (if you must eat a cheeseburger)
- Choose water as your beverage (if you must have a soda, choose diet)

BAJA FRESH MEXICAN GRILL

- Baja Burrito with half the rice
- Baja Ensalada with salsa verde dressing
- Fresh Mahi Mahi Ensalada
- Bean and cheese burrito
- Bean and cheese burrito; add grilled chicken
- Two Chicken Taco Chilitos
- Hold the sour cream; go light on the cheese and guacamole
- Choose water as your beverage (if you must have soda, choose diet)

SUBWAY

- Six-inch turkey, roast beef, chicken, or ham on whole-wheat bread or in a wrap
- Make your sandwich into a salad
- Skip the cheese or, if you must, go with Swiss cheese
- Add plenty of vegetables, such as tomatoes, pickles, black olives, cucumbers, and green peppers; go with spinach instead of iceberg lettuce
- Go light on the mayonnaise
- Drink water instead of soda

ANY PIZZERIA

- Choose a thin-crust vegetable, Hawaiian, or cheese pizza
- Add grilled chicken, ham, and veggies
- Do not order breadsticks
- Order a salad with low-fat dressing on the side

BOSTON MARKET

- Honey-glazed ham with steamed vegetable medley and fresh fruit
- Rotisserie turkey (without the skin) with green beans and fresh fruit
- Rotisserie chicken (without the skin) with garlic new potatoes and fresh fruit
- Asian chicken salad with half the dressing and no noodles
- Chicken or Turkey Carver with no sauce and fresh fruit
- Favor steamed veggies and garlic new potatoes as your sides
- Order water with your meal

TACO BELL

- Chicken soft tacos
- Bean burrito
- Chicken Burrito Supreme
- Fiesta chicken burrito
- Taco salad with salsa, and without the taco shell and tortilla strips
- Order any burrito or taco "Fresco Style" to decrease calorie and fat content by 25 percent
- Hold the sour cream; go light on the cheese and guacamole
- Choose water as your beverage (if you must have a soda, choose diet)

McDONALD'S

- Chicken McGrill sandwich with BBQ sauce instead of mayo, and a side salad with low-fat vinaigrette dressing

- Grilled chicken Caesar with ½ packet low-fat balsamic vinaigrette instead of Caesar dressing
- Grilled chicken California Cobb salad with ½ packet low-fat balsamic vinaigrette
- Cheeseburger (if you must) with a side salad topped with ½ packet low-fat balsamic vinaigrette
- Egg McMuffin
- Two scrambled eggs with an English muffin
- Fruit and yogurt parfait

CHIPOTLE MEXICAN GRILL OR MOE'S SOUTHWEST GRILL

- Instead of a burrito, skip the tortilla and order a bowl.
- Tell the server to go easy on the rice—one small scoop is enough. Decline the sour cream.
- Tell the server to go easy on cheese. If you order guacamole, have them put it on the side and split the order with a friend.
- Go to www.ChipotleFan.com to build your virtual burrito and calculate its nutrient value.

EATING OUT AT SIT-DOWN RESTAURANTS

- Choose grilled chicken or fish
- If ordering a steak, choose cuts with less marbling and trim off the fat
- Start with a salad with a low-fat dressing
- Choose steamed vegetables as sides
- Eat rolls and potato dishes in moderation

An overall lifestyle of healthy choices improves health and performance. Healthy eating habits overpower one not-so-great choice.

CORE WOMEN SUCCESS STORY

"I'm so much more aware of my body."

Denise Ciarcia • **Age: Thirty-nine** • **Hometown: Los Angeles, California**

Working as a set dresser in Hollywood, Denise Ciarcia is responsible for "dressing" a movie or television set in a hurry.

If an actor is pumping iron, it's Ciarcia's responsibility to make sure the weights are in place. If a television or sofa must be moved, Ciarcia must be ready to shoulder at least half of the load.

"I got tired of people saying, 'I'll get that for you,'" says Ciarcia (pronounced cee-R-cee-uh), who has worked on some of the biggest films and TV shows in the industry. "It wasn't just a matter of pride. I knew that if I couldn't hold my own, I wasn't going to get hired."

Ciarcia always has been thin, but she didn't always have a healthy physique. "I had no muscle and my skin hung really loose," she says. "No one would say that I was fat, but I wasn't fit either. Plus, I was really tight."

It didn't seem like much of a problem until her back went out. An MRI revealed a tear between the L-4 and L-5 vertebrae, which became an ongoing issue. One chiropractor prescribed an expensive program billed as "better than yoga and Pilates together."

Despite her effort and checkbook, Ciarcia's back kept giving out. Desperate for relief, she spotted a billboard for the Core Performance Center while driving around Santa Monica one afternoon. The facility, the first of Mark Verstegen's Core Performance Centers, provides a customized version of the Core Performance program in an upscale environment complete with the most modern training tools and on-site support.

Ciarcia embraced the program, learning the importance of firing her glutes, activating her hips, and keeping her tummy tight. She lost weight but found her new clothes were tighter in all of the right places. No longer did she have the gaunt "skinny fat" look she had endured for years.

Most important, her back stopped giving out. "I used to worry about throwing out my back leaning over to brush my teeth," Ciarcia says. "Now I'm constantly activating my core. I'm so much more aware of my body."

Working in the TV and film industry required some lifestyle adjustments. The cigarettes had to go, along with the late nights and drinking that often accompany smoking.

"I changed my outlook on what I do and where I eat," she says. "I like going to bed earlier and I no longer feel the need to go out all the time. This program has become my drug of choice."

The biggest challenge, Ciarcia says, is sticking to the Core Performance program when she's off shooting on location, sometimes for months. She recently was working in Michigan for two months during the winter and struggled to stick with her regimen. The crew was working seven days a week and she succumbed to poor nutritional choices.

She learned that preparing for such situations is vital. "If I'm going out of town now, I make sure I follow a workout from coreperformance.com. And there are healthier foods available on set. I mean, this is the film industry. We have a lot of people who work out and take care of themselves."

Ciarcia recently advanced to the role of property master, which is the head of her department. She has more responsibility now but is still ready to pitch in with set dressing.

Either way, she can tackle the heavy lifting.

CHAPTER 7 SUMMARY: Eating on the go presents a number of challenges. The key, once again, is proper planning. Stock your car, desk, briefcase, backpack, or diaper bag with healthy options so you won't have to turn to junk food when things get hectic. You need not eat poorly at sit-down restaurants. Go with grilled chicken or fish and steamed vegetables. If you must eat at a fast-food restaurant, make the best possible choice.

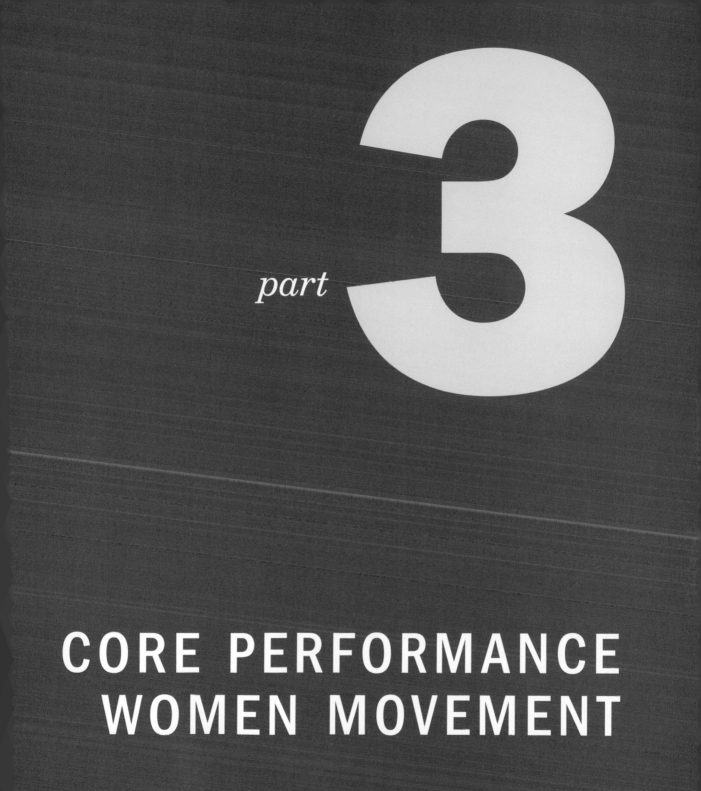

part

3

CORE PERFORMANCE
WOMEN MOVEMENT

A NEW REAR VIEW

love watching women move. That statement might get me in trouble with my wife, whom I *really* love watching move. What I mean to suggest is that women move with a combination of grace, fluidity, and confidence that men generally lack. When I watch women who are world-class athletes, executives, or household CEOs literally glide through life by properly using their God-given movement patterns, I marvel.

And confidence in motion is always attractive.

Unfortunately most women (and men), are incapable of executing proper movement patterns. They've lost the ability to use their core, this combination of shoulders, torso, and hips, to move in an efficient, powerful manner.

I spend a lot of time in airports and 90 percent of women I see hustling to and from flights have dysfunctional movement patterns. Few manage to use their gluteus maximus muscles (rear ends) as nature intended, to propel their hips forward.

This no doubt will come as a shock to those who work in the massive cottage industry devoted to helping women shape, tone, and otherwise sculpt their buttocks.

It's true, though. Even most elite female athletes who arrive at our Athletes' Performance training centers rarely activate their glutes. As a result, they never take full advantage of these tremendously powerful muscles that are built to go, not just for show.

That's because most of us—men and women—spend much of our time sitting on our glutes, which causes the muscles opposite them—the hip flexors—to become short and stiff, which prevent the glutes from firing.

Show me someone with tight hip flexors and I'll show you someone with a flat butt who has—or soon will have—back problems. Talk about adding insult to injury, or vice versa in this case.

Unless you reactivate your glutes, no buns-of-steel workout is going to make a difference. So take a moment right now and squeeze your left butt cheek, then your right. Imagine me making a pucker-up sound. Don't worry; I've done this for some of the biggest names in sports.

Congratulations. You now know how to activate your glutes. You'll want to do this throughout the Core Performance Women program as well as in routine daily activities such as walking, working, and climbing stairs.

There's nothing more powerful and attractive than a properly working set of gluteus maximus muscles. Who knew, right? Whenever you stare at someone's rear end, you're really appreciating that person's ability to develop their glutes through years of properly executed movement patterns.

If you take nothing else away from the Movement portion of the Core Performance Women system, remember this: It's all about the glutes. If you can learn to properly move through the hips and activate and fire your glutes constantly, you'll be well on your way to moving properly, giving your body stability, mobility, and a shot at a long-term, pain-free existence.

This does not just apply to women, though judging by late-night infomercials you'd think only the ladies have issues with their derrieres. Women now can buy underwear and panty hose with glute inserts. Plastic surgeons offer glute implants.

You'll save yourself that aggravation by following the Core Performance system. Not only that, you'll fight back against a technology-based society that put you in this predicament, with back pain, a hunched-over posture, and, of course, a flat butt.

Years ago ours was an agriculture-based society where most people used their glutes constantly. These days we still develop proper, natural movement patterns as children. Unfortunately the demands of the corporate cubicle culture, coupled with physical inactivity, take them away without us realizing it.

That's because the body is a phenomenal compensator. If there's pain or immobility in one area, a different region will pick up the slack, which can produce pain since joints and muscles designed for one task suddenly are overloaded.

The danger is what I call the "chain of pain." Those of us of a certain age remember the words from the song "Dry Bones," which we learned early in school or as part of a campfire sing-along.

The thighbone's connected to the hip bone. The hip bone's connected to the backbone. The backbone's connected to the shoulder bone . . .

This isn't just a catchy way to learn anatomy. It shows how everything in the body is connected, part of a kinetic chain. When part of the body is out of alignment, it's going to affect a different part, which affects another part, right up the line; thus the chain of pain.

Perhaps your body is out of alignment as a result of running or playing sports. Perhaps you don't engage in physical activity much at all. Your pain is a product of adulthood. As kids we move and function with what I call "perfect posture."

Perfect Posture

Perfect posture is the proper stance for optimal movement. Your shoulder blades should be pulled back and down, and your tummy should flat. If you're standing with perfect posture, your ears should be in line with your shoulders, your hips with your knees, and your knees with your ankles. If you're seated, there should be a straight line between your ears and hips.

Please take a moment and adjust your posture. Where I work we're often rushing around training athletes. But like any business, we must spend time at our desks. All of us make it a point to say "posture" when we're walking past a colleague and see her or him slouching. Some people even set their computer screen savers to show the word. It's a terrific reminder.

As adults we spend long hours hunched over a computer or steering wheel. We're wedged into airplane seats and are required to sit through long meetings. This disrupts the natural balance and alignment we developed as kids. We don't realize our shoulders are lurching forward, which places undue stress on our neck, hips, and back. We lose strength and flexibility while becoming sore in the joints.

Back pain is an epidemic, costing this country a fortune in medical costs and lost productivity. Back pain isn't an ailment so much as it is a symptom of other issues. When I see someone with back pain, I find that almost inevitably either one or both of their hip flexors—which attach to the thighbone and go through the abdominal cavity and attach to the lower part of the lower back—have become very restricted and tight. This pulls the pelvis and lower back into an anterior tilt, which causes back pain.

When one or both of your hip flexors is locked up, the body sends signals to the opposite muscles, shutting down the gluteus maximus muscles (or "glutes") and making the hamstrings less efficient. This creates a relationship where the hip flexors are dominant and the glutes are submissive. When you're out of balance in this dominant relationship, something is going to break down, and that's when you feel it in your back.

Let's take a closer look at this chain of pain. We could start anywhere, but let's return to that popular female trouble spot: your glutes. Glute pain is rare, though ironically the term "pain in the butt" is part of our everyday vernacular.

We spend most of our time sitting on our glutes, which causes the muscles opposite them—the hip flexors—to become tight. The neuromuscular relationship of these opposing muscle groups is known as *reciprocal inhibition*, which means that when one muscle group contracts, the opposite muscle relaxes to allow for fluid movement.

That's a good thing. Unfortunately when one area tightens up, its corresponding muscle group tends to shut down, creating poor movement patterns, and that leads to injury. The small muscles of the hips are constantly under pressure. One in particular is the gluteus medius. If not activated, it will lead to lower-back problems, knee pain, and groin strain. It's as if someone flipped the circuit breaker off, cutting off the power to these little muscles.

We're going to flip those circuit breakers on rapidly and efficiently to enable you to move properly, because the quality of your movement will play a significant role in the quality of your life. What is aging, really, but the loss of particular faculties and motor abilities? Our goal with *Core Performance Women* is to decrease pain, prevent further pain, and ultimately perform in the game of life, for as long as the game lasts.

Our goal in this section is to share some common injuries, ailments, and diseases that plague women specifically and find simple solutions.

Ankle injuries are painful in and of themselves, but they're notorious for launching this chain of pain. After an ankle sprain, the gluteus medius and gluteus maximus shut down, which tightens the hips.

People don't realize how dangerous it is to have tight hips. I cringe whenever I hear someone tell me that after a long period of inactivity, they've decided to take up running. If you have tight hips, you're going to be unable to move effectively. The force created by the pounding of running is stored in the muscles, tendons, and joints. If your hip capsule is locked down, it's as if a bone is welded to your pelvis—like having a cast on your hip. To get anything to move, you have to use excessive motion in your back and knees, and your thighbone is acting like a jackhammer to your knees. In the coming years, as baby boomers attempt to remain more active, you'll hear more about hip labral tears and the need for more hip replacements among the elderly.

Knees need to move up and down to create a balanced stride. When the legs are imbalanced because of tight hips, the knees go off track, causing cartilage to grind away at the kneecap. Knee problems also are a result of weak quadriceps, which often are being overpowered by tight hamstrings. Tight hamstrings arc a product of tight hips, which are a product of inactivated glutes. That's one reason hamstring strains and lower back pain are so commonplace. The chain of pain is relentless.

You don't have to take up running to experience this pain. Everyday life takes its toll. By sitting on our glutes all day, we're not just harming our lower body. That same endless sitting causes our shoulders to flex forward, giving us that hunched-over look. Not only that, we remain unconsciously in this position as we lift groceries or children, which produces pain in the shoulder, neck, and back.

Perhaps you have tennis elbow even though you've never picked up a racket. That's again because the body does such a terrific job of compensating. Instead of the shoulder supporting the movement—hence the term "shouldering the burden"—the elbow picks up the slack. Unfortunately the elbow wasn't meant for such heavy lifting and you feel pain.

Shoulder pain even hurts our appearance. Instead of standing tall, with our shoulder blades back and down, we become hunched forward and even shorter than we are. With our shoulders pulled forward out of balance, it's nearly impossible to be stabilized at the hips. And if we're not stabilized at the hips, well, the chain of pain just continues.

So there you have it, an updated rendition of "Dry Bones," the kinetic chain of pain produced by "dry" muscles and inactivity. The good news is that the muscles may shut down quickly, but it's just as easy to bring them back to life.

We started with Mindset in the first section of the book because, after all, it's necessary to get the mind right before embarking on the physical portion of the program. But in fact Movement is the foundation for Mindset. Movement is really the engine of your life since it improves cognitive function, relieves stress, and produces positive hormones that improve mental well-being. Movement also builds your immunity and makes you more resilient to illness and injury. It helps the body optimize its fueling; movement is the stimulus that allows the body to repair and rejuvenate itself several times in your life span.

If you're someone who has worked out before, you've no doubt experienced some of these benefits. You'll notice, however, that we use the word "Movement," not "exercise." *Exercise* has become a blanket term to refer to almost anything that does not involve sitting, including walking, jogging, gardening, and yard work.

Don't get me wrong; I'm a fan of any sort of exercise. But we want to think more in terms of using the proper movement patterns we were born with that we've lost as a result of sedentary, computer-based lifestyles. The idea is to get moving efficiently in an active lifestyle.

When it comes to movement, it's true that if you don't use it, you lose it. With today's technologically driven, sedentary lifestyles, more people are suffering from chronic dysfunctions and pain, which decrease the quality of their lives. That process can be reversed through proper movement training. It is the means for your body to heal itself, whether it's from the daily stresses of a normal or active lifestyle or the accumulation of stresses, as well as changes in your body over your lifetime.

The program that we've designed for you will address all stages of life, from the physically active periods of childhood and young adulthood to the more hectic stages involving career building and (for some) motherhood to menopause and the senior years.

In each stage the idea is to get you moving, especially if you're been living an inactive lifestyle. If you've been active, this will help you realign your body properly, especially if you've been dealing with chronic ailments and pain.

How are we going to fill such a tall order? By using a world-class game plan based on what we've used to support top female achievers, executives, and athletes. It will be organized in an easy-to-follow format that you can apply for the rest of your life. It's not a short-term solution but a proven, sustainable approach to a performance lifestyle.

Since the publication of our first book, *Core Performance,* in 2004, "core" training has become a popular buzzword. We're proud to see it become part of the American vernacular, with so many people applying it to their own high-performance lifestyles.

Unfortunately some have misappropriated Core Performance and its unique movement exercises to refer almost solely to washboard abs. Core Performance Movement has always been centered around Pillar Strength, an integrated system consisting of shoulder, torso (core), and hip stability.

That first book was embraced by men but even more so by women because women had a deeper appreciation for the seamless integration, depth, and intelligence behind this strategy, which wasn't overly clouded by testosterone and ego. Women from our Core Performance community have provided powerful insight as to how they used the program to overcome challenges to achieve things they never thought possible. That's helped us provide even more precise, female-specific solutions in this book.

Core Performance resonates with women because it provides the perfect focus. Women have been targeted with one group-fitness trend after another, when all they really want (though I hesitate to even suggest I know what women want!) is a simple yet powerful system of achieving optimal performance.

When we look at movement there's a tendency to put labels on various disciplines, such as yoga, Pilates, and their variations and insist people study and follow them instead of stepping back and recognizing that movement is the universal language we were born with; it's instilled in our DNA.

No longer must you feel confined to a particular discipline to give you parts of what you need. We're going to share with you the body's natural ability to move, tuned to your needs as a woman. That said, the Core Performance system will allow you to integrate your other passions, be they yoga, Pilates, or any other discipline.

When we talk about Movement, there are some core fundamentals you need to understand. Our goal is to create efficient software to operate your body. Unfortunately the majority of movement patterns have been infected with viruses from the demands of a fast-paced technological world and all of the other challenges of being a woman.

One of the limiting factors for women is stability. Of all the female athletes and achievers I've seen over the years, many have injury risks as a result of instability.

Stability refers to how your muscular system, specifically the smaller joint stabilizers, allows your body to hold itself in proper position at rest and even more so when it's moving. Stability plays a critical role in successful movement. If you lack stability, you increase the potential for injury, chronic pain, and overall movement inefficiency. That's not a path you want to go down.

The next part of the equation is mobility, your body's ability to go through active ranges of motion without creating tension. Mobility gives you fluid freedom of movement without creating unnecessary tension across joints. Together mobility and stability enable us to develop the right movement patterns and motor abilities, giving us physical skills that will enable us to live performance lifestyles regardless of which path we choose.

Efficient movement patterns empower us to live without pain and enjoy all of our pursuits with energy. One of the key tenets of the Core Performance system, unlike other programs influenced by bodybuilding, is that we're not training muscles or "body parts" but rather *movement patterns*.

Muscle is dumb; it's only as effective as what it's trained to do. It's part of your body's hardware. The Core Performance system is a software-driven approach to optimizing movement. We're reprogramming the software and working out the viruses, leaving you with long, lean, efficient "hardware."

Pillar Strength

One of the central tenets of the Core Performance system is the notion of Pillar Strength. Bodybuilding-based workout programs view the physique as a series of parts, and most people tend to think of movement as starting from the limbs. People adopt this same body-part mindset when they're in pain. They think their back pain isn't related to anything other than the back.

Actually movement starts from the very center of the body, the core area of the torso. That's why we refer to the torso as the pillar—its alignment and function directly correspond to the quality and efficiency of every movement. Everything is interrelated.

Pillar Strength is the foundation of all movement. It consists of hip, torso (or core), and shoulder stability. Those three areas give us a center axis from which to move. If you think of your body as a wheel, the pillar is the hub and the limbs are spokes.

There's a reason why parents are forever telling their children to sit up straight. With perfect posture you will significantly decrease the potential for injury in that chain of pain that starts with your lower back, descends all the way to your knees and ankles, and rises up to your shoulders, neck, and elbows.

Everything about the body's engineering is connected. What happens to the big toe affects the knees, the hips, and ultimately the shoulders. Many workout programs do more damage than good by producing muscle imbalances and inefficient movement patterns that sabotage the highly coordinated operating system we were born with.

Everything we do in this program will address the vital core areas of the hips, torso, and shoulders. When we can get them in proper alignment, building this Pillar Strength, we'll be well on our way to being pain free.

If you ever look at an anatomy book, you will notice that these three areas are woven together through an intricate figure eight that crosses your body from the left hip to the right shoulder and vice versa with muscular and fascial (connective) sheets that create the foundation for human movement.

Think of how movement evolves in infants. They move on their backs in a cross-crawl motion, using opposite arms and legs, until one day this action allows them to roll over, an innate movement. Soon they progress to pressing up, crawling, standing, squatting, and, finally balancing on one leg. At this point they begin stumbling and then advance into the efficient movement of walking. With each step they figure out how to stabilize their bodies. This makes them smile; moving is fun, after all.

Aging reverses that process. Inefficient movement is painful, no fun at all. Many women lose the ability to squat and maintain their balance, tightening and weakening and creating poor posture. Eventually they lose the ability to stand, surrendering the core fundamental movement patterns they developed as toddlers. But instead of conceding that devolution is an unavoidable part of aging, why not look at getting older as a process of taking these movements to new levels? In this program you're going to take your body to the highest levels of performance and movement capabilities by challenging yourself to increase flexibility and stability. We'll help you do this by adding resistance or increasing the balance demands. This will put you further and further away from the regression of aging.

Think of this process of taking an active role in your long-term movement patterns as "pro-hab." Unlike "re-hab," a reactive process that responds to an injury suffered, pre-hab is a process of protecting your body from backsliding into the pain, inactivity, and dysfunction that lead to your downward spiral.

If you can master the following three elements of Pillar Strength—hip stability, core stability, and shoulder stability—both while working out and in everyday movement, you will go a long way toward a healthier life.

Hip Stability

Hip stability may be the number-one issue facing women when it comes to injuries and ailments. Injuries of the anterior cruciate ligament (ACL) of the knee have reached epidemic proportions among young women, and not just athletes. Nobody can pinpoint a reason, with theories ranging from the increased physical nature of women's sports to biomechanical issues to a possible tie-in to menstrual cycles.

ACL injuries lead to other knee problems, along with shin splints, stress fractures, and other injuries. ACL injuries often are related to a lack of stability and mobility in the hips; the knee moves to compensate for the hip.

The hip cuff is the control unit for your lower body. It governs the thigh, which interacts with your knee and affects your foot position. The centrality of the hip cuff is why tremendous attention must be paid to strengthening the muscles in and around the area, as they are critical in controlling everything below your hips and everything above as well.

The hip cuff consists of more than forty muscles in and around your lower pelvis that are responsible for much of your lower-body movement. Even if you think you already have the ultimate hip-and-glute workout routine, I assure you that you haven't come close to addressing this key area.

Hips are the most overlooked area when it comes to decreasing the potential for injury. Most back and hip problems occur because of improper mobility and stability and faulty utilization of the hips. Most people are locked down or unstable in their hips. If one of your hip capsules is locked down, it's as if one of your thighbones is welded to your pelvis—imagine wearing a permanent cast on your hip. To get anything to move, you would have to use excessive motion in your knees and back to make up for your hip's immobility. The lower and middle back share some common responsibilities with your hips, but they were meant to be secondary, not primary, initiators of movement. By maximizing efficiency in and around the hip cuff through improved mobility, stability, and strength, you will discover the engine that will propel you throughout daily life, to say nothing of creating "buns of steel."

As I mentioned at the beginning of this chapter, we want to focus on becoming glute dominant instead of quad dominant. This is a key concept. Most women move from their knee joints rather than their hip joints; they're "quad dominant." Their knees move first, stimulating the quadriceps muscles to fire at the onset of movement. This is a dangerous thing because the hub of your wheel is your pelvic area—not the quads. You want to absorb force through the more powerful center of your body toward your glutes, which will enable the limbs to work together to produce force. To try to absorb this much force in the quads alone is to invite ACL and other leg injuries.

Imagine if you slip on a patch of ice. If your knees and quads move first, you're probably going to fall, likely resulting in a knee injury. But if you can absorb that force through the center of your body and your glutes, you're less likely to tumble and if you do, it's less likely to produce a knee injury.

The reason women tend to be quad dominant is that they have a larger "Q angle," the angle at which the femur (upper leg bone) meets the tibia (lower leg bone). Women's hips are slightly wider relative to their knees and often a woman's knees fall more toward the midline of the body, creating a greater angle from the knee to the hip.

This is the price women have to pay for being able to produce the miracle of childbirth. There's nothing we can do to change this, obviously. But what you can do is be aware of it so that when you look in the mirror or watch your workout routine, your knees are not coming together or rubbing together.

This program will help you develop more femoral control by focusing not on your knees but on your hip cuff, which is the control center for both your knees and lower legs. We'll spend lots of time on movements that challenge the hip rotators. These exercises might feel like butt busters but they are actually knee and back protectors, designed to give your body the ability to control the angles and better disperse force into your muscular system.

Core Stability

Core stability is much more than a chiseled midsection or washboard abs. The core consists of the muscles of your torso, primarily your abdominals and lower back. It's the vital link between hip and shoulder stability, and it includes such muscle groups as the rectus abdominis, transverse abdominis, internal and external obliques, erector spinae, latissimus dorsi (lats), and many small stabilizing muscles between the vertebrae of the spine known as the multifidi.

The multifidi are the tiny muscles that often get shut off because of a back injury and never become reactivated, causing long-term back problems. These muscles cannot function alone; you have to help them by training your core muscles to become strong and stable, with the right types of recruitment patterns that will enable them to work in tandem with your shoulders and hips.

Instead of just focusing on the abs, we want to create the framework for all movement. The aim isn't just a well-sculpted midsection; it's a high-performance core. In order to maximize the benefit of the exercises in this book, it's important to keep your tummy tight, not just while exercising but all day. Think of your tummy flat against the hip bones. Keep your tummy tight, as if pulling your belly button off your belt buckle. This isn't the same as sucking in your gut and holding your breath. Keep the abdominals in, but still breathe.

Your abdominal and lower back muscles work as a team. The point guard is the transverse abdominis, which is the first muscle that's recruited each time you move. If you can keep your "TA" activated and your tummy tight, you'll be well on your way to efficient movement and preventing long-term deterioration. With this program it will work into your subconscious and become automatic.

Shoulder Stability

We tend to think of the hands and arms as carrying the workload for the upper body, but it's really the shoulders that should bear or "shoulder" that weight.

Most of us don't realize how hunched over we are from sitting at computers, traveling in cars and airplanes, and carrying backpacks and briefcases. People tend to think that this affects only the elderly, but that's not the case. The next time you're people-watching, pay attention to the position of people's thumbs. If they're rotated in, pointing toward the centerline of the body, chances are their heads and shoulders have rotated forward—or soon will.

Unless those people do something, I guarantee that they soon will have rotator cuff, back, and neck problems, which will limit their ability to participate in the daily activities of life.

This is often an issue with taller women, especially those who hit a growth spurt at a young age. They feel awkward since they haven't grown into their bodies and look different from their friends. They haven't yet realized what an advantage height can be in life. So what do they do? They subconsciously slouch over to make themselves appear shorter so they don't stand out in the crowd. They end up with pain in their neck, lower back, and shoulders because their posture is so flexed forward.

Our natural instinct is to drop the shoulders forward, especially after long periods of sitting. But you ought to do the opposite: Elevate your sternum and let your shoulder blades hang back and down, which will give you proper posture. Imagine yourself "feeling tall," as if there's a fishhook inserted under the sternum, pulling us up.

CORE WOMEN SUCCESS STORY

"I had tried everything."

Pauletta Washington • **Hometown: Los Angeles**

Pauletta Washington spent more than two decades as a workout warrior. From boxing to boot camps, spinning to Pilates, cross-training to bodybuilding, she mastered them all. A typical workout was ninety minutes, and two hours was not uncommon.

She figured she'd get better results from training longer and harder, especially as she got older. She juggled training sessions around her busy life as a mother, professional musician, and member of several boards and committees. She brought intensity to all of her endeavors, especially to her group fitness classes, where in recent years she could keep up with women twenty years younger.

By most measuring sticks Washington was a picture of health and fitness. Unfortunately the pounding of years of marathon workout sessions had left her with painful flare-ups in her back and knee.

"I'd take time off and get better and then they'd flare up again," Washington says. "It was like hitting a brick wall. Instead of making progress, it was a digression. It was extremely frustrating because working out was such a part of my life and I was wondering what I was going to be able to do. I had tried everything."

She had all but resigned herself to a life with chronic pain when she was introduced to the Core Performance program through the Core Performance Center in Santa Monica, California. There she embarked on a program geared toward creating core strength and eliminating the pain in her knee and back. Best of all, her training sessions were less than an hour.

Washington, who was accustomed to spending much longer in the gym, was skeptical. How could she obtain such results in so little time?

"I'm so booked sometimes, and with this program I can get a full workout and still be able to do all of what I have to do," she says. "I don't have to sacrifice anything."

The painful flare-ups of the back and knee are a thing of the past. "Not only that, but I seem to be becoming a lot stronger in those areas and have more stamina," she says.

Having embraced most every fitness craze of the last decade, Washington is thrilled to be following a program that can sustain her for life.

"That's what excites me the most," she says. "When I was doing classes, I always knew that it couldn't last. I could maintain the intensity, but I started feeling broken down and it was taking longer to recover. I look at younger women doing the things I used to do and I think, 'It's just a matter of time.' With this program it doesn't have to be that way. You really can get stronger as you get older."

The exercises in this program will require you to bring your shoulders back and down, but you'll want to make it a daily habit. To make lasting change, you must lengthen your "internal rotators" (chest and lats) and strengthen the "external rotators," the muscles of the upper back, rotator cuff, and the rest of the shoulders.

This posture is the exact opposite of the shoulder shrug, the motion you make when you say, "I don't know." If you make a habit of bringing your shoulders down—think of dropping your shoulder blades into your back pocket—you'll be amazed at the results. People will find you more confident and think you've lost weight because you're no longer slouched over. They might even think you've grown.

How is that possible? Think about it. You probably know someone, perhaps a grandmother or elderly friend, who is not as tall as she used to be. Age and perhaps osteoporosis have pulled her head and neck forward, giving her a permanent hunched-over appearance. At that point there's not much that can be done for her.

But if you're a younger woman, it's not too late. Without realizing it you may have lost a quarter to a half inch by slumping over. By bringing your shoulder blades back and down, as well as improving hip and core stability, you'll get that height back. More important, you'll appear more confident and dynamic, as if you're gliding through life like the successful woman you are.

CHAPTER 8 SUMMARY: Pillar strength, the foundation of movement, consists of shoulder, torso (core), and hip stability and strength. Effective workouts train the body for functional everyday movement. It's about training movements, not body parts. Make it a daily habit to "feel tall," bringing your shoulders back and down as if you're dropping them in your back pockets. Keep your tummy tight, and fire those glutes.

THE CORE PERFORMANCE WOMEN WORKOUT: AN INTRODUCTION

The multibillion-dollar health and beauty industry is fueled by the endless quest of women to look younger. Research of the aging process suggests that while we might not be able to live decades longer by taking care of our bodies, we can dramatically improve the quality of our remaining years.

That's a key part of the Core Performance philosophy: It's not just about the length of time; it's about the *quality* of our time. This program arrests the natural decline of aging. It *could* allow you to live longer, especially if you entered the program in poor condition. It definitely will provide a higher quality of life for however many years you enjoy.

But unless you take action now, you're not only ensuring this decline, you're expediting the process. I'm sure you know women, perhaps friends or relatives, between the relatively young ages of thirty-five and fifty-five who say it hurts to get in and out of a car. They avoid squatting because it hurts their knees and back. It's sad because instead of being vibrant, happy, pain-free women they've aged long before their time.

Women (and men) spend so much time, effort, and money on plastic surgery in an attempt to roll back time on parts of their body where it's impossible to beat Mother Nature. I'm not about to pass judgment on folks who make these decisions, but I'd suggest that they could discover a cheaper, more effective fountain of youth of sorts by mastering the Core Fundamentals of this program.

It all starts with the notion of activating your core. You want to keep your shoulders relaxed, hanging back and down, and your tummy tight. You also want to initiate movement from your hips and glutes.

If you suffer from back or joint pain, do not exercise regularly, and possess a lack of energy and muscle tightness, the principles of Core Performance Women will get you out of the rut. These are the same principles applied at Athletes' Performance to improve and prolong the careers of professional athletes.

This program was designed to be an effective and efficient solution for the woman with a hectic life. The goal is to make the most of the limited time you will commit and provide a huge return on investment, thus improving the quality of your life now and for the rest of your life.

A common downfall of many fitness programs is a lack of progression: People do the same exercises until their bodies are so used to the program that the exercises no longer confer any benefit. Or they're required to spend more time—time that they don't have. The great thing about Core Performance Women is that you'll spend less time as you become more proficient in the movements. This allows you to add more

Equipment List

We've kept the equipment list as simple as possible. If you're someone who likes to work out at home, a set of dumbbells that can be adjusted for different weight is ideal and takes up less space than dumbbells of varying weight. A cable pulley station is something you probably won't invest in for home use. If you're not in a gym, these movements can be done without a pulley station. Everything else is compact and mobile.

_____ 1. Pair of dumbbells

_____ 2. Bench

_____ 3. Cable pulley station

_____ 4. Mini band

_____ 5. Foam roll

_____ 6. Pair of slides

_____ 7. Tennis balls (2)

_____ 8. Blue Thera-Band pad (a rolled-up gym towel works just as well)

_____ 9. Heart rate monitor

advanced movements or additional reps without increasing the amount of time you've committed.

It's no different than any other skill set. The more you develop a skill, the more efficient you can be at it. There are many home improvement tasks I could tackle, but there's no way I'd ever be half as efficient as the contractor who performs them every day.

You can customize the workout schedule to fit your busy schedule. You might want to invest in a home gym to save time commuting to the gym. Instead of paying monthly gym fees, take that money and assemble your own compact Core

Performance Center in a corner of your home by visiting the Core Store at www.coreperformance.com.

The versatile, inexpensive pieces of equipment you'll use in this program don't take up a large amount of space. We've also engineered this system to adapt and grow with your needs. Recognizing that there will be times when you're limited by a lack of equipment, we've provided options. Here then, are the first four units of the Core Performance for Women workout. (The fifth, Regeneration, warrants its own chapter.)

Pillar Prep

As discussed in the last chapter, Pillar Strength is the foundation of all movement, consisting of hip, torso (or core), and shoulder stability. Those three areas give us a center axis from which to move. Traditional workout programs think of warm-ups in terms of activating the legs or arms. But since movement starts from the pillar, it makes sense instead to first warm up the pillar. That's the role of Pillar Prep; it's simply the activation of your shoulders, torso, and hips.

Pillar Prep is a brief series of movements that activates and strengthens the pillar, giving our bodies great stability and efficiency prior to doing other movement patterns. We want to make sure everything is turned on and activated prior to going through any further movement. By activating the shoulders, torso, and hips, you'll be much better prepared to go through Movement Preparation, Strength/Power, and Energy System Development (ESD). Pillar Prep sets the physiological and psychological stage to incorporate Pillar Strength into every movement of your workout, since every exercise or movement pattern requires it. Pillar Prep allows us to spend a few focused minutes getting our minds and muscles tuned in to what we're about to do. Pillar Prep activates both your body and mind to focus on the power of your pillar in every upcoming movement.

Movement Preparation

One thing that's made our Core Performance system so well-received is Movement Preparation or "Movement Prep." Movement Prep was engineered to address the majority of injuries and ailments associated with movement and help you perform at a higher level.

Movement Prep is a series of movements that help boot up your body just like the software in your computer. How you warm up can significantly enhance the quality of your performance.

Likewise an improper warm-up, which might include only traditional static stretching, actually shuts muscles down rather than turning them on. This can compromise the effort you put into the workout. Most warm-ups are a waste of your precious time.

You might be under the impression that hopping on a stationary bike for five or ten minutes prior to a workout is no big deal, but it's ineffective in that it minimizes your return on investment for that workout.

Your time and effort are valuable to us, so let's look at the so-called warm-up in terms of numbers. If you spend ten minutes a day, five to six days a week for forty-eight weeks, over the course of a year that's two straight days of training you've devoted, equivalent to a pair of twenty-four-hour races.

If you spend that time on a stationary bike, you'll get little return. But by mastering Movement Prep and incorporating it into your day, you will experience dramatic physical changes while decreasing and preventing pain. That in turn will help you perform better.

Movement Prep might look like a combination of active Pilates and yoga blended together in a fluid, integrated way. That's true, but it also will activate all of the small stabilizing muscles in your body that assist with balance. It provides an incredible bang for your buck, and I know you'll love it.

The foundation of Movement Prep is making sure you're always maintaining great

Pillar Strength, which is a workout in itself but also lengthening and strengthening the muscles in each movement pattern. This is why we start with Pillar Prep to wake up and turn on your pillar power.

Movement Prep, which I've used with elite athletes for nearly two decades, is an active series of warm-up exercises that efficiently increases the core temperature; activates the nervous system; lengthens, strengthens, stabilizes, and balances muscles; and, as the name suggests, prepares you to optimize the upcoming movement. Movement Prep will reestablish the mobility, coordination, and joint stability you enjoyed in your younger years and improve your strength, balance, and coordination—in other words it will heighten your body's ability to process information.

You want to improve the long-term mobility and flexibility of your muscles. Rather than have them stretch and revert to where they were—as is the case with stretch-and-hold routines—you want your body to remember these new ranges of motion.

This is done through a process of lengthening the muscle (known as active elongation), which is more effective than a traditional stretch. Here's the crucial difference: You don't just stretch your muscles and let them snap back into place like a rubber band. Instead you show your muscles how to use the motion.

Movement Prep will be a challenge at first. Just remember that the top champions in sports have struggled with it just as much. Like you, they shared the mindset that they soon would master it, whether it would be in a day or week.

Movement Prep is a powerful self-evaluation tool. As you go through it and master the movement patterns, pay attention to your posture and pillar strength. Also be aware of any asymmetries between your right and left sides, as well as your front and back. As you get deeper into the Core Performance system, Movement Prep will be a daily diagnostic of where your body is and will help you focus on areas you need to address.

Strength/Power

Women often have a resistance to resistance training, what some might call weight training or strength training. That's understandable. After all much of what you read and hear is that resistance training is going to make you big and bulky.

This simply is not true. Women lack the testosterone needed to put on the type of muscle that's unattractive. If you've come across women in the gym or in magazines who have *waaay* too much muscle, they're probably bodybuilders or figure/fitness models who have been taking steroids or other harmful supplements. So how do you avoid this kind of bulk? Don't take this junk. It's that simple.

Not only do bodybuilders create an unattractive look, they're not necessarily becoming stronger, which is our goal.

Instead of focusing on isolated muscles, the cornerstone of the bodybuilding-based programs, we're going to focus on creating better stability and mobility throughout your core region, which in turn will make you stronger when you perform the movements of everyday life. The goal of bodybuilding is to build big muscles, increasing their size, a process called hypertrophy. You probably have an image of a female bodybuilder who technically looks like a woman but who probably is hormonally enhanced and, in some respects, has moved toward being a man!

This obviously is not normal. The power of this system is that we're going to be training integrated movement patterns, which simply are greater challenges to existing movements that you use every day—or at least you used to as a kid.

This is why your body, regardless of how strong and powerful you become, regardless of how much wattage your body can produce and how much weight you lift, will still look very natural, athletic, and fluid. It will be the ideal picture of what the female body looks and moves like. You can work as hard as you want in the Core Performance system and you will not develop massive, thick, short, stiff muscles.

One of the primary goals of the Core Performance system is to decrease your body fat while maintaining and improving the efficiency of your lean body mass. Lean mass is so much more valuable than massive bodybuilder muscle because it optimizes its performance, mobility, stability, movement patterns, power, strength, and endurance.

The Power/Strength training unit will look familiar because it's an integration of the movement patterns that we've been mastering with the foundation of Pillar Strength and of Movement Prep. We're simply making them more challenging by adding resistance or increased stabilizing demands, much like you would with Pilates.

You'll also notice that most of these movement patterns force you to use the right side independent of the left, the front independent of the back and with rotational movements so we create a balanced body working in harmony.

You may notice an emphasis on your body's posterior chain (backside) and on working to make those muscles strong and powerful, which will improve your posture and help you meet the physical demands of being a woman.

We do the majority of our work in a circuit-type fashion, which means we alternate these movement patterns into pushing movements (upper and lower body), pulling movements (upper and lower body), and rotational movements.

As with everything in the Core Performance system, this helps us accomplish our goal of getting the most accomplished in the least amount of time. If we do an upper-body press exercise, the muscles become fatigued. That's a good thing, of course. Now if we follow that up immediately with an upper-body or lower-body pull exercise, we're allowing those muscles that performed the upper-body press to rest briefly. By going right into an opposing exercise, those resting muscles will experience an "active stretch" that facilitates the muscle's recovery. So we've improved the quality and the quantity of the program and will get results faster.

Not only that, we're increasing our workout density, the amount of work per unit of time. We're not resting, just alternating movement patterns to make the most of our time. If you've spent any time in a gym, you've probably noticed people who do one set of an exercise, then wait between thirty seconds and two minutes before attempting another set of the same exercise.

By training so efficiently, we're working the cardiovascular system as well as the muscular system. Much like interval training, this will stress the body and stimulate its adaptation to stress while decreasing body fat, increasing caloric expenditure, and improving overall performance levels for hours and days after the workout.

You'll gain power and strength as we continually challenge you by increasing the number of sets and/or repetitions, by increasing the resistance, and also by adjusting the tempo in which you perform each rep.

Tempo simply refers to the cadence in which you go through each movement pattern. An example of this would be if I give you a cadence of 3-2-1, you will lower the weight in three seconds, pause at the isometric position for two seconds, and then press the weight up in one second, hence a 3-2-1 tempo for eccentric (lowering), isometric (bottom), and concentric (raising) contractions.

We're going to teach you to explosively move and contract your muscles, which is critical in everything from athletics to protecting yourself from injury as you age. The term often used for this is plyometrics, the idea of your muscle acting as a spring, efficiently storing and releasing energy.

This ability is as critical for someone who wants to run a 5K race or participate in sports as it is for a woman trying to catch herself from slipping on a patch of ice. It improves your body's ability to store and recycle energy into the next movement.

It's important to remember that injuries often occur when we are tired, whether in sports or daily life. Conditioning is not just a function of your lungs, but possessing efficient movement patterns, greater relative power and strength (pound for pound), and elasticity that leaves you feeling constantly fresh.

These efficient movement patterns will help you avoid trauma-producing energy leaks. Energy leaks occur when your body tries to produce force, such as when your foot hits the ground while walking and running. The energy goes up your leg into the rest of your body and finds an area of instability, perhaps around a hip. There the energy dissipates or "leaks" into this unstable joint, creating greater trauma on the joint and surrounding connective and muscular tissue. That leads to more than 70 percent of chronic pain and injury.

With the Core Performance system, we'll eradicate energy leaks by improving efficiency with these movement patterns.

Energy System Development (ESD)

What's the first thing that comes to mind when you hear the term "cardio"? You probably think of running at a slow pace—"slogging"—on a treadmill, pedaling on a stationary bike, stepping on an elliptical machine, or some combination of all of them. You're moving at a steady pace, never really challenging yourself.

If you've spent any time in a gym, you're familiar with the "cardio queen." This is the gal who hops from cardio machine to group fitness class, never touching a dumbbell. She's all about burning more calories than she takes in, a losing battle if ever there was one. Worst of all, she's spending an awful lot of time—hours per day in some cases—fighting this losing battle.

This entire Core Performance Women system, especially the Strength/Power portion, is geared for you to create more lean mass, which will burn more calories at work and at rest. Your body becomes a leaner fat-burning machine.

As for cardio, there's an important place for it in this program, but let's take a moment and redefine it. We no longer want to think of cardio as the preferred activity of the cardio queen, who puts forth so much effort and gets precious little return on investment. This complete steady-state approach to cardio training leads to plateaus, which discourage people in the pursuit of their goals. It just doesn't cut it.

Not only is such training a waste of time, it actually could be inviting pain and dysfunction in your body. Much like driving a car without proper wheel alignment is going to result in major repairs, the practice of undergoing long, repetitive training—even at a slow, steady pace—could result in serious injuries.

There's nothing wrong with the word *cardio*, which is short for *cardiovascular*, which means "of, relating to, or involving the heart and the blood vessels." Unfortunately it's come to be associated with long, slow, nonefficient training.

That's why we refer to this section of the program as Energy System Development, or ESD. Many women embark on cardio activity because they want to lose weight. Others fall into that false mindset of "not wanting to get big" and avoid strength training. Yet others want to lower their risk of cardiovascular disease, which is a noble goal.

The purpose of our cardiovascular system is to pump blood—cardio work is meant to improve the system. What is the value of creating greater cardio endurance? For athletes it's the ability to play sports like basketball or soccer. Endurance allows us to make efficient, high-speed movements for short bursts of time followed by an active recovery, followed by another intense burst of movement.

Now think of the average gym-goer, aimlessly "working out" on the treadmill or bike while talking on the cell phone or watching CNN. You don't need much endurance for that kind of work.

In order to get the most out of our energy systems, we need to have a purpose. That purpose should be improving the body's ability to use energy, improving the fuel efficiency for the type of activity that you do.

This is not going to require just one long, slow, steady-state "workout" that numbs your neuromuscular system and creates repetitive trauma. This will require more energy and focus—but likely less time—to give you a greater return on investment.

We're going to ask you to do various lengths of interval training. There will be intense bouts of effort followed by decreased amounts to allow your body to recover.

By alternating intervals of work and rest, you'll burn more calories during the session, and the best part is that your body will continue burning them long after you're

CORE WOMEN SUCCESS STORY

"Core strength will make the difference."

Vicky Arthur • Age: Eighteen • Hometown: Kensington, Maryland

Vicky Arthur was a thirteen-year-old eighth grader when she received a copy of the original *Core Performance* book in 2004.

Back then her sport of choice was rock climbing and she competed at a high level across the country. The Core Performance program helped her create the stability and mobility needed to excel in a demanding sport that requires both.

As she advanced to high school, her focus turned to team sports and field hockey, where core conditioning was equally important.

"Your quads, hamstrings, and glutes take a beating in field hockey, and if you don't have that core stability, you're not going to be very good," she says. "You won't be able to hit and shoot and you're not going to be able to avoid defensive tackles, as we call them in field hockey. In terms of importance in the sport, core strength is second only to your overall ability and technique."

Like many teenagers, Vicky does not spend much time thinking about what she eats, if only because she's not the one purchasing groceries. Thankfully her parents have instilled in her some healthy eating habits

done as it tries to play catch-up. It's a gift that keeps on giving. Previously you might have done thirty to sixty minutes of cardio without feeling much of an impact. Now you might feel exhausted after fifteen to twenty-five minutes of ESD training. You'll get twice the benefit in half the time.

This is not going to be easy, but I guarantee it will be effective and rewarding. When you are in a position to efficiently expend energy and set personal records session after session, avoiding plateaus and continuing on an upward spiral of success, it will that will prepare her for college. There she'll likely avoid the notorious "freshman fifteen," the extra pounds young women pack on once left on their own to eat for the first time.

Having attended an all-girls high school, Vicky is well aware of the eating issues young women face.

"As an athlete, I'm fortunate to be around a group of girls who understand the idea of food as fuel," she says. "But I see other girls who are not involved with sports constantly changing diets and worrying about body issues. Some of them are dealing with eating disorders, and you wonder if it will get worse once they get to college. I feel like I'm prepared to make the right decisions."

Vicky is proud to be an early adopter of the Core Performance system, which has helped her thrive in both high school and club field hockey. One of her club team's trainers recently showed the team a copy of *Core Performance* and mentioned they'd be doing some of the exercises. Vicky already was up to speed, having used the program to improve her game and attract scholarship offers from major Division I programs. She signed to play at the University of Connecticut.

"A program like Core Performance is so important because when I head off to play Division I sports, everyone is going to be at the top level of what I saw in high school and beyond," she said. "Everyone will have good technique. Core strength will make the difference."

be so empowering and motivating that it might become your favorite part of the Core Performance system. Intervals require some effort, but you can bet it will be effort infused with intelligence that efficiently moves you toward your goals.

In order to do this efficiently, we're going to need to establish three simple target heart rate zones, which we can later tune as you reach higher levels of performance. This is far from an exact science, but let's get started by taking 220 minus your age to establish your maximum heart rate.

If you've been riding the bike for years or jogging on the treadmill but have seen little change in your body composition, you will be in for a surprise. Like the elite athletes that come to our training centers, you will soon see that ESD training will produce the most rapid improvements in less time.

The benefit of the entire Core Performance Women system, including the nutrition program, is about performance and feeling better in the daily game of life, but it's also about dramatic change in your body. If you stick with the program, you'll have less body fat and more lean mass. Some of this will be apparent immediately because of the changes in your posture, but much of it will be a combination of ESD and following the nutrition plan. Even if you haven't lost scale weight, you'll have more lean body mass and people will ask if you've dropped a few pounds.

In this section we're going to develop three energy systems: the alactate, lactate, and aerobic. The *alactate* system refers to your body's ability to do high-level work for periods of up to twelve seconds. Your body's *lactate* system refers to its capacity to do high-intensity work for up to three minutes. The *aerobic* system is your body's ability to work beyond three minutes.

With intervals, intensity is more important than time. You're going to maintain the same amount of time—twenty-five minutes—throughout the program, but you'll ratchet up the intensity as you go along.

The smaller the ratio of work to rest, the more you will improve your body's anaerobic/ventilatory threshold—which means you've increased your body's ability to do hard work. With anaerobic exercise the body relies more on energy stores than it does on oxygen. It puts you in oxygen debt, which increases the burning sensation in muscles and makes the body compensate to get your heart rate to come back down.

But there's tremendous benefit to this. It's like tuning a high-performance engine—in this case, the lungs, heart, and related systems. Interval training increases energy production in every cell and in the highways to those cells, allowing you to burn energy more efficiently.

The best part about ESD is that it won't take long. I'm not going to ask you to go out and jog—or slog—for three to five miles. Gym equipment provides an effective cardio workout. Jump aboard a bike, treadmill, elliptical trainer, or VersaClimber and set it on manual. Make use of the machine's heart rate monitor or, preferably, use your own (as discussed earlier in the equipment section). But don't feel limited to gym machines. Feel free, especially if you're enjoying great weather, to do your ESD training outdoors, whether it's by sprinting on a track, running stadium stairs, or climbing hills in your neighborhood. One of the great attractions of training is getting outside, so if you'd prefer to be outside doing your ESD work rather than laboring in a health club, by all means go for it.

Whenever you decide to do your intervals, don't forget form. Don't undermine your hard work with sloppiness in movement patterns or in sloppy running mechanics. It's counterproductive. Focus on keeping both feet pointing straight ahead. Fire your glutes and quads, and don't forget to use your arms. You will be amazed at how much more fluid you feel, and at the amount of speed you can maintain with less effort.

Each ESD workout starts with a warm-up period. Then you'll alternate intervals of work with intervals of recovery. You'll do between one and three repetitions of this interval, depending on the stage of the program, followed by a cool-down period, for a session lasting between twenty-one and thirty minutes.

You will notice that ESD includes intervals of work and recovery; we call this the work-to-rest ratio. The greater the rest, the higher quality the work should be. The lower the ratio—for instance, one second of rest per one second of work (one-to-one)—the bigger the challenge, since the body has less time to recover. That increases your capacity to do work.

CHAPTER 9 SUMMARY: The Core Performance for Women workout is an integrated program that trains the body for lifelong movement. It consists of four components: Pillar Prep, Movement Preparation, Strength/Power, and Energy System Development (ESD). Pillar Prep activates and strengthens the hips, torso (or core), and shoulders before you do other movement patterns. Movement Prep increases core temperature and lengthens and strengthens muscles, reinforcing proper movement patterns so that you make long-term flexibility and stability gains. The Strength/Power unit helps you build strength and produce force through resistance exercises. Such training, contrary to popular belief, does not "make you big" but rather creates lean, beautiful, fat-burning muscle. Unlike traditional, laborious cardio work, ESD focuses on quality, not quantity, and it improves the function of your cardiovascular system while building endurance and helping your body create new energy levels.

CORE PERFORMANCE MOVEMENTS

The goal of this program is not to keep you in the gym for hours but to provide you a sizable return on a modest investment of time in the form of better performance and overall health. This is not a quick-fix, twelve-week system, but the foundation of your active life.

The Core Performance Women workouts are classified into three categories: Strength, Endurance, and Regeneration. In the Strength and Endurance routines, you will do a series of exercises from the Pillar Prep, Movement Preparation, and Strength/Power units, followed by Regeneration. The organization of these units will provide you the maximum flexibility in planning your week, getting the most results in three to four days a week and allowing you to integrate your favorite classes (Pilates, yoga, spin, etc.) or sports activities (hiking, running, stick-and-ball sports, etc.).

We've created a flexible program that allows you to plan for each week regardless of how busy it may become. Each workout will take no more than forty-five minutes. The workout days fall into three categories: Strength, Endurance, and Regeneration. When laying out your schedule, just remember that you should not have more than two combined Strength/Endurance days without scheduling a Regeneration day.

If, for instance, you wish to train on Mondays, Wednesdays, and Fridays only, you could do a Strength workout on Monday, an Endurance workout on Wednesday, and return to Strength on Friday. The following week, do two Endurance days and one Strength day. If you'd like to train on Monday, Tuesday, and Thursday, you could do Strength on Monday, Endurance on Tuesday, and Strength on Thursday.

If you would like to train six days a week, terrific. Just remember to work in a Regeneration day after every two days. So if you do Strength on Monday and Endurance on Tuesday, schedule a Regeneration day for Wednesday.

Below are three ways you might organize your week depending on your schedule:

OPTION	MON	TUES	WED	THURS	FRI	SAT	SUN
A	Strength	End	Regen	Strength	End	Regen	
B	End	Strength	Regen	End	Strength	Regen	
C		End	Strength	Regen	Strength	End	Regen

The Regeneration days can include the specific Regeneration exercises that we'll discuss more in the next chapter, or it may simply be a day in which you enjoy Pilates, yoga, swimming, or your favorite sport. The goal is to restore your system physically and psychologically after two challenging days. So relax and have fun. Think about how you can recover and decrease the overall stress in your life from the time you wake up until the time you go to bed. Use some of the specific Regeneration strategies we've laid out in Chapter 12 as well as the very specific routines to decrease and prevent pain. We're giving you both a general recovery strategy but some specific solutions as well. If you notice any particular issues, such as foot pain or upper back trouble, you'll find a solution for that trouble spot.

The difference between the Strength workout days and Endurance workout days is that on the Strength days you will do some exercises from the Strength/Power unit and on the Endurance days you will do twenty to twenty-five minutes of Energy System Development (ESD) work.

Within each workout—Strength or Endurance—there are three levels. Level 1 helps lay the foundation for your long-term success. The goal here is to master the movements while also gaining strength. You'll note at the beginning of each level, we're only asking you to do one set of each exercise, and we know that you'll feel that there's more than enough time to do this. Please take this time, especially in the early stages, to ensure that you're doing the movements properly. Examine the illustrations in this book or check out the videos at www.coreperformance.com.

The goal is to master the subtleties of each movement. Be in tune with your posture and body alignment. Make sure the proper muscles are firing. Take note of your natural weak spots and areas you'll want to focus on as this becomes a true workout in the later stages. As you work through the program, moving to Level 2, you will do a more advanced, slightly different variation or what we call a progression. You might add two movements together or go from using both legs to one, for instance.

The other way we challenge you is by increasing the density, the amount of quality work you do in a given amount of time, which is the ultimate definition of fitness. Early on it might take you ten minutes to complete the Pillar Prep and Movement Preparation exercises. Later on it might take you only five minutes.

We not only have designed these challenging workouts to improve your fitness but

CORE WOMEN SUCCESS STORY

"Even more motivation."

Jaclyn Wynn • **Age: Thirty-one** • **Hometown: Fountain Hills, Arizona**

Jaclyn Wynn has a unique perspective on the Core Performance program, having demonstrated the movements for years as a model for DVDs, online at www.coreperformance .com, and for Core Performance books, including this one.

Wynn played soccer in college at Arizona State and professionally for the Boston Breakers of the now-defunct WUSA. Not bad for a young woman whom doctors once believed would battle health issues.

At the age of five Wynn was diagnosed with a genetic condition that predisposed her to having high cholesterol. Doctors prescribed medications, but when Wynn's mother balked, they suggested she place her daughter on a program of diet and exercise.

Jaclyn dabbled in a variety of sports growing up, gravitating toward soccer and gymnastics. After college she trained for the WUSA at Athletes' Performance alongside soccer great Mia Hamm.

The league lasted just three seasons and Wynn eventually landed back at Athletes' Performance, working in sales and marketing for the company's various consumer products. She maintained her competitive athlete mindset, competing in two Olympic-distance triathlons.

"I can see how people get away from training once their competitive careers are over, whether that's high school or later," Wynn says. "They get into the work world and priorities change. I knew with soccer over, I needed something else to keep me active. I had never biked seriously, barely had swum, and so it was definitely a challenge."

The bigger challenge came when she got pregnant a month after her second triathlon, early in 2008. Wynn knows she's one of those people other women envy, having lost all thirty-five pounds of pregnancy weight within eight weeks of giving birth in 2009.

She points out that she's no genetic freak—indeed, predisposed to having high cholesterol—and though the weight was the same, her body composition was way off. She posed for this book just seven weeks after childbirth, flattered to be asked sight unseen. Any quick rebound, she says, is due to following the Core Performance program up until two days before going into labor.

"I continued to do Movement Prep, basically everything but not using much weight, if any," Wynn said. "Doctors told me that if you're in good shape going in, then the delivery is generally much easier. I don't quite believe that; the birth itself was the worst experience of my life. But I definitely believe the recovery process was very easy and quick because of following this system prior to and during pregnancy."

Like a lot of new parents, Wynn and her husband, Jason, found dealing with their new daughter, Cameron to be exhausting, especially during those first weeks of parenthood.

"Jason complains that he hasn't worked out in three weeks and his energy level has dropped," Wynn says. "I feel the same way. Getting even thirty minutes three times a week just boosts your energy level so much."

Not only did Wynn face the adjustment to motherhood, but also stay-at-home motherhood, leaving the workforce at the age of thirty-one. It's not an unusual pattern for women of her generation, spending a decade establishing a career only to give it up to raise children.

Wynn is thankful and excited to be a stay-at-home mom, but she admits feeling a little guilty at a time when women are held to a different standard, all but expected to juggle a full-time career and motherhood. Even the logistics seem daunting. Having to deal with a breast pump during the two-day photo shoot for this book, she developed a new appreciation for women who return to work while still breast-feeding.

"I don't know how those women do it," she says. "It wasn't an easy decision to leave my job, especially because I love what I do and the people I worked with. The baby is my first priority. I definitely think down the road I'd like to pick up a career again. But I understand now the dilemma this is for women."

She and Cameron have taken some Mommy and Me yoga classes. Usually she's hard-pressed to get in a fifteen-minute workout at home, though with Daddy watching Cameron she manages to spend as much as ninety minutes in her garage going through the Core Performance program. She plans to finish another triathlon long before Cameron's first birthday.

"Staying with this program really helps my motivation and energy level," Wynn says. "Once you have someone else to care for, you have even more motivation to stay in shape, and when you do, that makes you happier and you feel better inside and out. Not only that, you need all the energy you can get. This program gives me the support I need."

also to meet the challenge of fitting into your hectic schedule. The workout time will always be forty-five minutes on Strength days and forty-five minutes on Endurance days. But you'll progressively get more done within those forty-five minutes.

Within each level of each unit (Pillar Prep, Movement Prep, Strength/Power, ESD, Regeneration), there are four stages: A, B, C, and D. Stage A is the learning stage where you might not break a *physical* sweat, but you will be mentally challenged as you learn these new movements. Once you master them, you will add more sets and reps in Stage B. Once you're able to complete these sets and reps in the given time, you will have earned the right to advance to Stage C, which gives you more to do in the same time, and yet again in Stage D.

After that you will have mastered enough—and be fit enough—for the next level. We will repeat this process with Level 2. Here you will notice that while the exercises are similar, they are harder and you will be asked to get more done in less time.

How is this possible? For starters, we're working at a brisk pace. The reason most people spend so much time in the gym—or think that it's necessary—is because they never improve their workout density. They add more reps, sets, and exercises, but because they work at a slow, plodding pace, it takes more time. We're not going to do that.

The other reason you're able to accomplish more in the same amount of time is that you're becoming more efficient. Have you ever prepared to give a speech or talk? If so, you've probably noticed that the more you practice, the shorter the talk becomes. It's not necessarily because you're talking faster or truncating parts, but you're becoming more comfortable with what you're saying. You might find that you can pack more into that thirty-minute talk than you thought.

The same philosophy holds true for this workout. As you get more comfortable, you work more efficiently.

Level 3 consists of a pair of Core Challenges. One of the greatest challenges of sticking to a program is being on the road, away from your normal routines. These two simple, efficient routines work on any travel schedule, anywhere in the world, and let you keep your high levels of fitness with limited time, space, equipment, and energy.

You might also undertake the Core Challenges for the opposite reason. Perhaps after a hectic period of travel and other stresses you have a stretch of several weeks where your life is back to some semblance of normalcy. You can use the Core Challenges, which are more intense, to create your own "boot camp" and inspire you to eat clean and properly.

The great thing about the Core Challenges is they're designed and can be further tweaked to meet those seemingly contradictory demands. You can truncate the program for use on the road and make it more difficult for those times you're home for extended periods of time and ready to push your limits.

Core Workout Specifics

Let's take a look at the specifics of the two workout days: Strength and Endurance. You will start with ten minutes of Pillar Prep, where you'll activate and develop your

Pillar Strength through movements that both isolate and integrate the shoulders, torso, and hips. Since Pillar Strength is the foundation of all movement, it's crucial that we begin our workout by creating this base for the workout and the rest of the day.

After Pillar Prep, you will spend ten minutes on Movement Preparation, where you'll lengthen and strengthen your muscles and get your body ready for the rest of the workout. Next you'll proceed into twenty-five minutes of Strength/Power training, which will include many of the same exercises from the Movement Prep unit, as well as a few new ones. Here we have combined some challenging upper body pressing and pulling movements, along with some lower body pressing and pulling. In Levels 2 and 3 we add some exercises that focus on a combination of speed, power, and endurance.

At the end of forty-five-minute Endurance days and the Level 3 Strength days, there is a Regeneration unit. I promised to keep these sessions to forty-five minutes, and I will. There are parts of this workout program that include five to ten minutes of Regeneration within the forty-five minutes. But whether your workout day includes a designated Regeneration block or not, I want you to think of Regeneration as something that works its way into your entire day. The Regeneration unit has specific solutions for recovery and relieving pain or spasms. But it's also a lifestyle strategy that includes getting the proper nutrition after your workout, along with finding ways to recover throughout the day.

Like Strength days, Endurance days begin with Pillar Prep and Movement Preparation. In order to improve your stability, mobility, and overall form we will continue to emphasize these movements to make them stronger and more efficient. After this, you will spend twenty minutes in Level 1 and twenty-five minutes in Level 2 on some targeted Energy System Development (ESD).

With ESD, you're going to use your newfound power and efficient movement patterns with every step, glide, revolution, and stroke you take. Pay close attention to the amount of work and the amount of rest in each interval. Once you start to feel everything come together, don't be scared to start stepping on the accelerator; your body will respond. Admittedly it can be scary to go where you haven't been before. Don't worry; you'll be rewarded with results.

CHAPTER 10 SUMMARY: The Core Performance Women workout is categorized into Strength, Endurance, and Regeneration days. The workouts consist of combinations of five exercise units: Pillar Prep, Movement Preparation, Strength/Power, ESD, and Regeneration. Within each Strength and Endurance workout day, there are three levels, never taking you more than forty-five minutes total (see Appendix).

CORE PERFORMANCE WOMEN EXERCISES

B efore we organize our workouts into Strength, Endurance, and Regeneration days, let's take a unit-by-unit look at each exercise. Some of these exercises may seem awkward or difficult at first, but don't worry—you'll adapt quickly. One of the exciting parts of the Core Performance Women program is experiencing "aha" moments as you discover new methods of improving performance.

Pillar Prep exercises are on pages 169–184. You'll find Movement Prep moves on pages 185–200. Strength/Power exercises begin on page 201 and run through page 223. The Regeneration section runs from page 224 to page 236.

PILLAR PREP

Mini Band External Rotation

STARTING POSITION
Stand in a quarter squat with your feet just wider than your hips and a mini band above your knees.

PROCEDURE
Keeping your left leg stationary, rotate your right knee in and out for the prescribed number of reps (see Appendix). Then switch legs and repeat.

COACHING KEY
Keep both feet flat on the ground and your pelvis stable. Don't let the knee of your stationary leg drop in.

YOU SHOULD FEEL IT
Working your glutes.

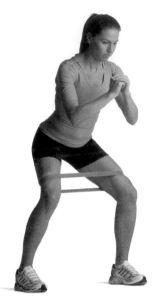

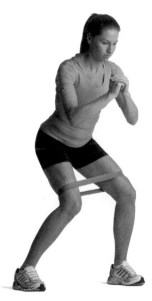

Mini Band Bent Leg Walk

STARTING POSITION

Stand in a quarter-squat position with your feet hip-width apart and a mini band above your knees.

PROCEDURE

Walk forward with small steps as alternating elbows drive back with each step. Continue for the prescribed number of reps on each foot.

COACHING KEY

Keep your chest up and maintain your back's natural arch. Keep your knees pushed apart and over your toes at all times. Keep tension on the mini band at all times.

YOU SHOULD FEEL IT

Working your glutes.

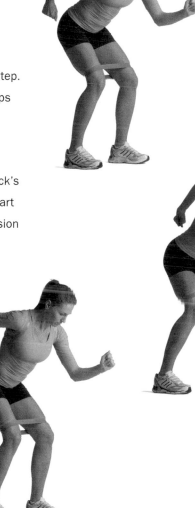

Squat—Mini Band

STARTING POSITION

Stand with your arms at your sides, your feet shoulder-width apart and pointing straight ahead, and a mini band around and above your knees.

PROCEDURE

Maintain perfect posture and initiate movement with your hips. As you reach your arms far forward, push your hips back and down until your thighs are parallel to the floor. Return to a standing position by pushing through your hips. Keep your knees out. Repeat until you've completed all your reps.

COACHING KEY

Keep your knees behind your toes during the movement. Also, push your knees out against the band so that they do not collapse to the inside during the movement. If you extend your arms in front of you, you can sit back more comfortably. Keep your chest up and maintain your back's natural arch.

YOU SHOULD FEEL IT

In your glutes, hamstrings, and quads.

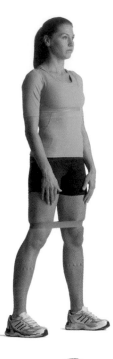

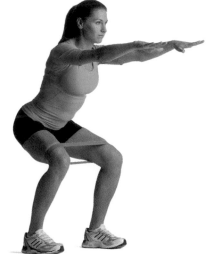

Overhead Squat—Mini Band

STARTING POSITION

Stand with your arms straight up in the air, your feet shoulder-width apart and pointing straight ahead, and a mini band around and above your knees.

PROCEDURE

Maintain perfect posture and initiate movement with your hips. Keeping your arms up, squat your hips back and down until your thighs are parallel to the floor. Return to a standing position by pushing through your hips. Keep your knees out. Repeat until you've completed all your reps.

COACHING KEY

Keep your knees behind your toes during the movement. Also, push your knees out against the band so they do not collapse to the inside during the movement. Keep your chest up and maintain your back's natural arch. Keep your hands over your feet.

YOU SHOULD FEEL IT

In your glutes, hamstrings, and quads.

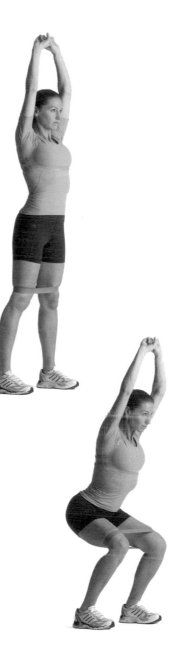

L–To Press–Bent Over

STARTING POSITION

Stand hinged over at the waist with your back flat and your chest up.

PROCEDURE

Glide your shoulder blades back and down, lift your elbows to the ceiling as they bend to 90 degrees, and rotate your hands toward the ceiling, and press them over your head. Reverse to the starting position and continue for the prescribed number of reps.

COACHING KEY

Initiate the movement with your shoulder blades, not your arms.

YOU SHOULD FEEL IT

Working your shoulders and your upper and lower back.

Foam Roll—Thoracic Spine

STARTING POSITION

Lie faceup on the ground with your knees
bent and heels on the ground with a foam roll
under your midback and your head supported
with your hands. Keep your elbows together.

PROCEDURE

Roll from the middle of your back up to your
shoulders and repeat for 30 to 60 seconds.

COACHING KEY

Hold your hands behind your head with your
elbows pointed to the sky and close together.
Hold on sore sports for 30 to 60 seconds.

YOU SHOULD FEEL

As if you were getting
a deep massage.

Thoracic Spine Mobility

STARTING POSITION

Tape two tennis balls together with athletic tape to form a peanut shape. Lie on your back, knees bent and heels on the ground, with the balls under your spine just above your lower back and your hands behind your head.

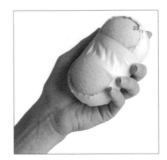

PROCEDURE

Perform 5 crunches, then raise your arms over your chest and alternately reach over your head for 5 repetitions with each arm. Move the balls up your spine for 1 to 2 inches and repeat the crunches and arm reaches. Continue moving the balls up your spine until they are just above your shoulder blades and below the base of your neck.

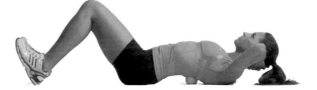

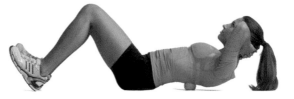

COACHING KEY

During the crunches, try to "hinge" on the ball rather than roll over it. Think about keeping your ribs pushed down toward the ground during the arm reaches.

YOU SHOULD FEEL

As if you were getting a deep massage in your mid- to upper back.

Plank—Kneeling with Shoulder Tap

STARTING POSITION

From a kneeling push-up position, raise one hand to the opposite shoulder. Hold for 1 to 2 seconds. Return and switch sides. Repeat for the prescribed number of reps.

COACHING KEY

Keep both knees on the floor and do not move your back.

YOU SHOULD FEEL IT

Working your torso.

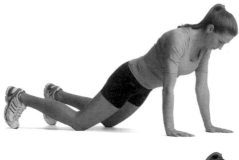

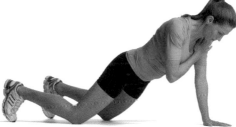

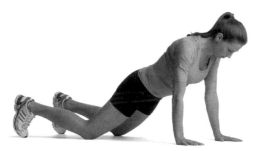

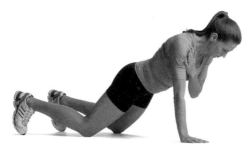

Pillar Bridge—Diagonal Arm Lift

STARTING POSITION

Assume a push-up position with your forearms on the ground and your feet wider than shoulder-width apart.

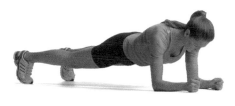

PROCEDURE

Without moving your torso, lift your right arm up and slightly to the right and hold for 1 to 2 seconds. Return to the starting position and repeat with your left arm. Repeat for the prescribed number of reps.

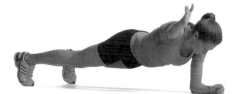

COACHING KEY

Try to keep your weight even on both feet as your arm lifts. Do not let your trunk move as your arm leaves the ground. Keep your stomach tight throughout the movement.

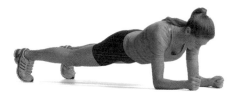

YOU SHOULD FEEL IT

Working your shoulders and trunk.

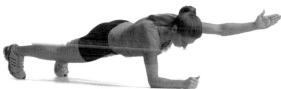

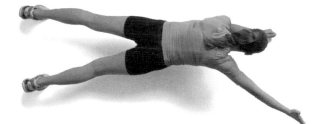

Y's—Floor

STARTING POSITION

Lie facedown on the floor with your bent arms raised slightly above shoulder height, to create a Y with your torso and thumbs up.

PROCEDURE

Glide your shoulder blades toward your spine and lift your arms off the ground. Return to the starting position and repeat for the prescribed number of reps.

COACHING KEY

Keep your stomach tight and your thumbs up. Move from the scapulae (shoulder blades), extending your shoulders and hands.

YOU SHOULD FEEL IT

Working your shoulders and upper back.

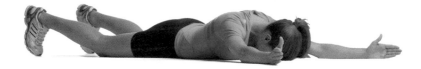

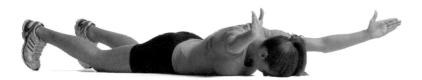

Glute Bridge—Marching Hip Flexion

STARTING POSITION

Lie faceup on the ground with your arms
to your sides, your knees bent, and your
heels on the ground.

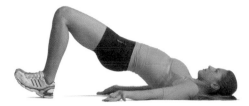

PROCEDURE

Lift your hips off the ground until your knees,
hips, and shoulders are in a straight line.
Hold the position while lifting your right knee
to your chest. Return your foot to the ground
and repeat with your left knee. Continue for
the prescribed number of reps.

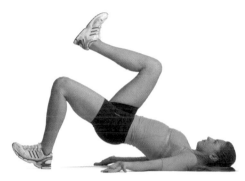

COACHING KEY

Do not let your back hyperextend. Do not
let your hips drop as your knee comes to
your chest.

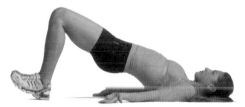

YOU SHOULD FEEL IT

Working mainly your glutes, and secondarily
your hamstrings and lower back.

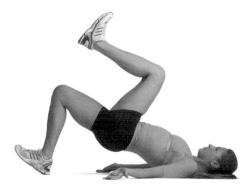

Lateral Pillar Bridge with Pec Stretch

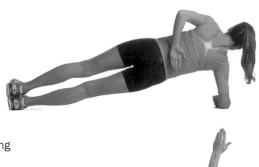

STARTING POSITION

Lie on your side with your body in a straight line and your elbow under your shoulder, feet stacked, your top hand behind your back, palm facing out.

PROCEDURE

Sweep the top hand over your head, keeping it as long as possible until your palm is facing behind you. Complete the prescribed number of reps. Switch sides.

COACHING KEY

Reach as far as you can during the sweep and keep your hips up and pushed forward.

YOU SHOULD FEEL IT

Working the shoulders, torso, and lateral hip stabilizers. You also should feel a stretch in the pec and shoulder of the arm you're moving.

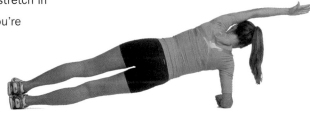

Glute Bridge—Knee Extension with Adduction

STARTING POSITION

Lie faceup on the ground with your arms to your sides, your knees bent, and your heels on the ground. Place a blue pad between your knees.

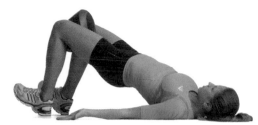

PROCEDURE

Lift your hips off the ground until your knees, hips, and shoulders are in a straight line. Hold the position while extending your right knee. Return your foot to the ground and repeat with your left knee. Repeat for the prescribed number of reps.

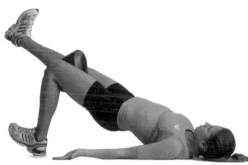

COACHING KEY

Don't let your back hyperextend. Don't let your hips drop as your knee extends.

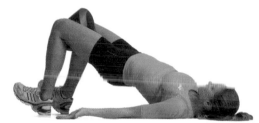

YOU SHOULD FEEL IT

Working your glutes mostly and to a lesser degree your hamstrings and lower back.

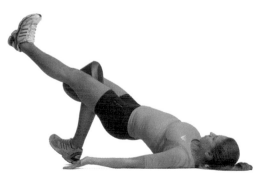

Lateral Pillar Bridge—Marching

STARTING POSITION

Lie on your side with your body in a straight
line and your elbow under your shoulder,
your feet staggered. Push your hip off the
ground, creating a straight line from
ankle to shoulder.

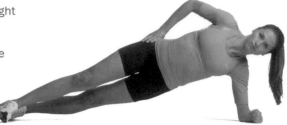

PROCEDURE

Lift your bottom knee to your chest, hold for
1 to 2 seconds, and return. Lift the top knee
to the chest, hold for 1 to 2 seconds, and
return. Complete the prescribed number
of reps. Switch sides.

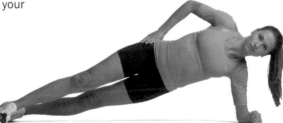

COACHING KEY

Keep your hips up and forward. Don't let your
back move throughout the movement.

YOU SHOULD FEEL IT

Working the hips, shoulders, and torso.

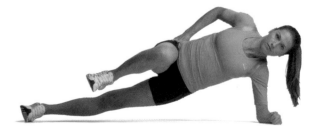

MOVEMENT PREPARATION

Lateral Squat

STARTING POSITION

Stand with your feet just outside your shoulders.

PROCEDURE

Shift your hips to the right and down by bending your right knee and keeping your left leg straight. Your feet should be pointing straight ahead and flat on the ground. Push through your right hip, returning to the starting position. Then shift your hips to the left and down by bending your left knee and keeping your right leg straight. Continue, alternating sides, for the prescribed number of repetitions.

COACHING KEY

Keep your knee on your "working side" behind your toes. Keep your opposite leg straight, your back flat, and your chest up.

YOU SHOULD FEEL

A lengthening and stretching of your glutes, groin, hamstrings, and quads.

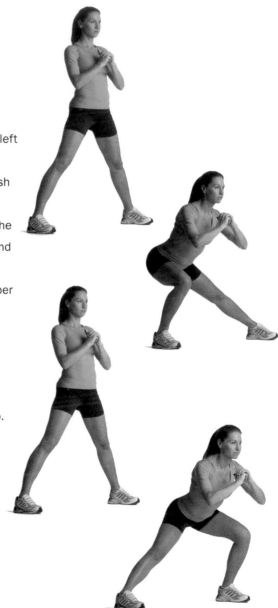

Lateral Lunge to Drop Lunge

STARTING POSITION

Stand with your feet wider than shoulder-width apart.

PROCEDURE

Shift your hips to the right and down by bending your right knee and keeping your left leg straight. Your feet should be straight ahead and flat on the ground. Push through your right hip, returning to the starting position. Next, reach your right foot 2 feet behind your left foot. Square your hips back to the starting position, and sit back and down into a squat. Return to the starting

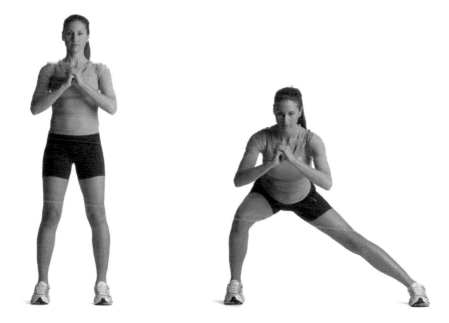

position and repeat on the other side. Repeat
for the prescribed number of reps.

COACHING KEY

For the lateral lunge, keep your knee on your
"working" side behind your toes. Keep your
opposite leg straight, your back flat, and
your chest up. For the drop lunge, maintain
your weight on the heel of your front leg.

YOU SHOULD FEEL

A lengthening and strengthening of your
glutes, groin, hamstrings, and quads.

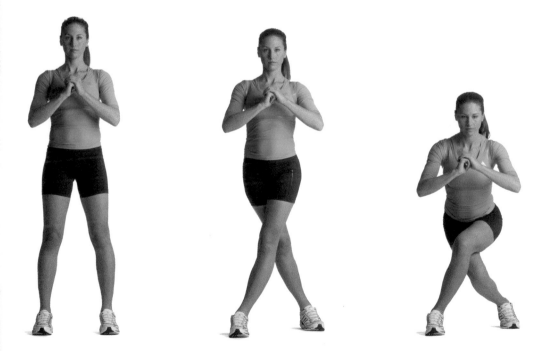

Inverted Hamstring to T Hip Mobility

STARTING POSITION

Stand on your left leg with perfect posture, your left arm holding a chair or other support, your shoulder blades back and down.

PROCEDURE

With your standing knee slightly bent, keeping a straight line between your ear and ankle, hinge at the hip and elevate your right leg behind you. Rotate your pelvis and shoulders up, feeling a stretch on the inside of your standing thigh. Return to the "T" position, stand, and repeat for prescribed number of reps. Repeat on the other side.

COACHING KEY

Move your shoulders and hips as one unit. Keep the leg you're standing on slightly bent at the knee and keep your back leg lifted toward the sky throughout the movement.

YOU SHOULD FEEL

Stretching on the inside of the hip you're standing on, as well as stretching your hamstrings and challenging your balance.

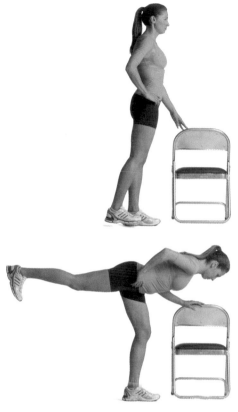

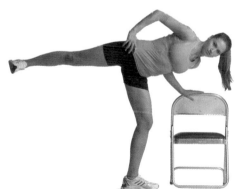

Inverted Hamstring with Reach

STARTING POSITION

Stand on your left leg with perfect posture.

PROCEDURE

Keeping a straight line between the ear and ankle, hinge over at the hip and elevate your right leg behind you. Reach forward with both arms. When you feel a stretch in your hamstring, return to the starting position by contracting your glute and hamstring. Repeat the movement, alternating legs for the prescribed number of reps.

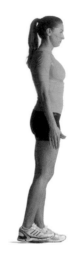

COACHING KEY

Keep the knee of the leg you are standing on slightly bent. Keep your back flat and your hips, legs, and arms parallel to the ground. Maintain a straight line from your ear through your hip, knee, and ankle of your leg in the air. Try not to let your raised foot touch the ground between repetitions.

YOU SHOULD FEEL IT

Stretching your hamstrings and challenging your balance.

Knee Hug (in place)

STARTING POSITION

Stand with your back straight and your arms at your sides.

PROCEDURE

Lift your right knee to your chest and grab below the knee with your hands. Pull your right knee as close to your chest as you can while contracting your left glute. Return to the starting position and repeat on the other side. Continue, alternating sides, for the prescribed number of reps.

COACHING KEY

Keep your chest up. Contract the glute of the leg you are standing on.

YOU SHOULD FEEL

A stretch in the glute and hamstring of your front leg and in the hip flexor of your back leg.

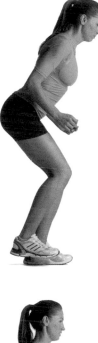

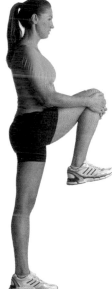

Knee Hug (moving)

STARTING POSITION

Stand with your knees bent, back straight, and arms at your sides.

PROCEDURE

Lift your right foot off the ground and squat back and down while standing on your left leg. Lift your right knee to your chest and grab below the knee with your hands. Pull your right knee as close as you can to your chest while contracting your left glute. Step forward and repeat on the other side. Continue alternating sides and moving forward for the prescribed number of reps.

COACHING KEY

Keep your chest up. Contract the glute of the leg you are standing on. Do not let your knee slide forward during the squat.

YOU SHOULD FEEL IT

Stretching the glute and hamstring of your front leg and the hip flexor of your back leg.

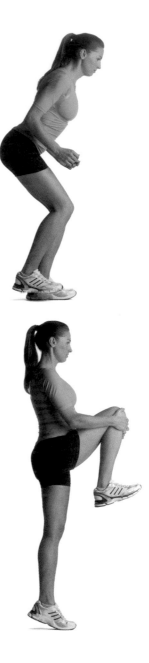

Handwalk

STARTING POSITION

Hinge at the waist and walk your feet out into a push-up position.

PROCEDURE

Raise your hips into a downward dog yoga position. Hold for 1 to 2 seconds and walk back to standing position. Complete the prescribed number of reps.

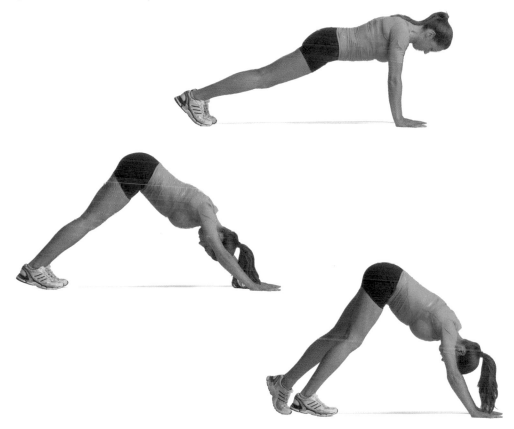

COACHING KEY

Keep your knees straight and your stomach tight.

YOU SHOULD FEEL

A stretch in your hamstrings, lower back, glutes, and calves.

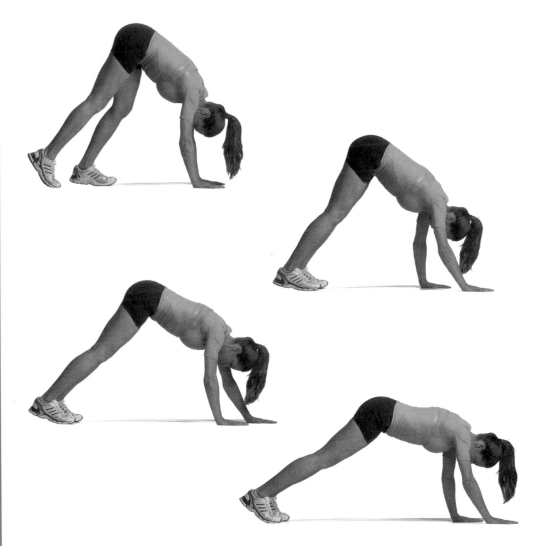

Handwalk with Arm Lift

STARTING POSITION

Hinge at the waist and walk your feet out into
a push-up position.

PROCEDURE

Raise your hips into a downward dog yoga
position. Lift one arm and hold for 1 to 2
seconds, then the other. Complete
the prescribed number of reps.
Walk back to standing position.

COACHING KEY

Keep your knees straight and your
stomach tight.

YOU SHOULD FEEL

A stretch in your hamstrings, lower back,
glutes, and calves.

Forward Lunge, Elbow to Instep + Rotation (in place)

STARTING POSITION

Stand with your back straight and your arms at your sides.

PROCEDURE

Step forward into a lunge with your right foot. Place your left hand on the ground and your right elbow to the inside of your right foot, and hold the stretch for 1 to 2 seconds. Rotate your right arm and chest to the sky as far as you can. Hold for 1 to 2 seconds. Take your elbow back and down toward your instep and reach through to your opposite side. Place your right hand outside your foot and push your hips to the sky. Return your right elbow to the inside of your right foot and repeat for the prescribed number of repetitions on each side.

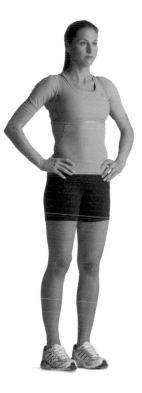

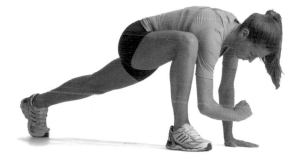

COACHING KEY

Keep your back knee off the ground. Contract your back glute during the stretch.

YOU SHOULD FEEL

A stretch in your groin, your back leg hip flexor, and your front leg glute and hamstring.

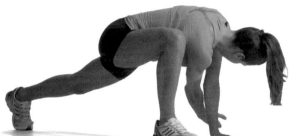

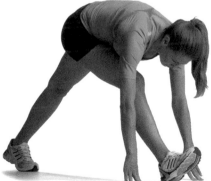

Forward Lunge, Elbow to Instep + Rotation (moving)

STARTING POSITION

Stand with your back straight and your arms at your sides.

PROCEDURE

Step forward into a lunge with your right foot. Place your left hand on the ground and your right elbow to the inside of your right foot, and hold the stretch for 1 to 2 seconds. Rotate your right arm and chest to the sky as far as you can. Hold for 1 to 2 seconds. Take your elbow back and down toward your instep and reach through to your opposite side. Place your right hand outside your foot and push your hips to the sky. Finally, step forward into the next lunge. Repeat for the prescribed number of repetitions on each side.

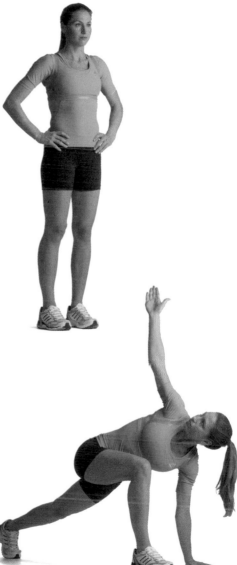

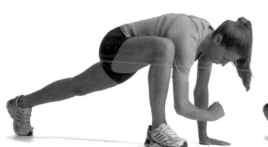

COACHING KEY

Keep your back knee off the ground. Contract
your back glute during the stretch.

YOU SHOULD FEEL

A stretch in your groin, your back leg hip
flexor, and your front leg glute and hamstring.

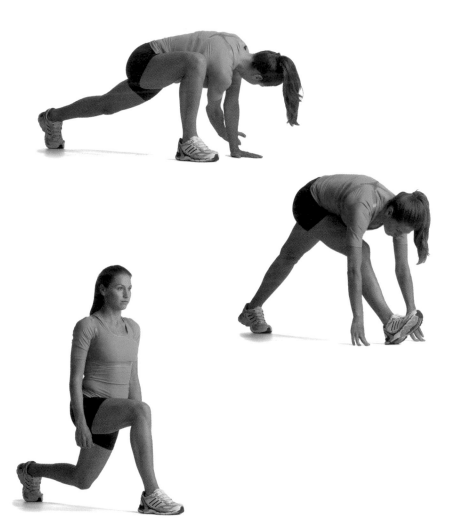

STRENGTH/POWER

Bent-Over Row—Alternating Dumbbell

STARTING POSITION

Hinge over at your hips, back flat, holding a pair of dumbbells at your sides in a row position.

PROCEDURE

Lower one arm as far away as you can without rotating your back and return to the start position. Lower the other arm. Repeat for the prescribed number of reps.

COACHING KEY

Keep your back flat and don't let both hands be in the down position at the same time.

YOU SHOULD FEEL

A stretch in your back. This is a strength movement for your back.

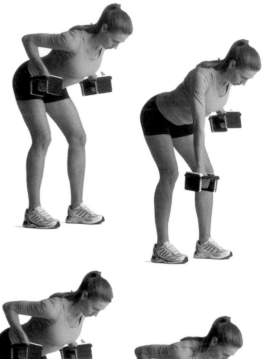

Bent-Over Row—1 Arm, 1 Leg Dumbbell

STARTING POSITION

Stand on your right leg, hinged over at the waist, holding a dumbbell with your right hand and holding on to a stable, waist-high surface with your left hand. Lift your left leg to form a T with your body.

PROCEDURE

Slide your right shoulder blade toward your spine and then lift the weight to your body by driving your elbow to the ceiling. Return to the starting position and repeat for the prescribed number of repetitions, then switch sides.

COACHING KEY

Move with your shoulder, not your arm, to initiate the row. Keep your back level—your shoulders should stay parallel to the floor—and fire the glute of your extended leg to keep it parallel to the floor. Extend the leg on the same side of the hand doing the lifting. Keep your knee slightly bent.

YOU SHOULD FEEL IT

In your back, lats, and shoulders.

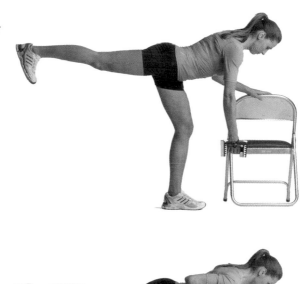

Reverse Lunge—Dumbbell (slide)

STARTING POSITION

Stand on a carpet with one foot on a slide, such as a file folder, or on a hardwood floor with one foot on a towel.

PROCEDURE

Slide your foot backward and drop your hips toward the ground by bending your front knee without letting your back knee touch the ground. Return to the starting position by pushing up with your front leg. Continue for the prescribed number of repetitions, then switch legs.

COACHING KEY

Do not let your front knee slide forward past your toes or collapse to the inside. Keep your chest up. Keep the glute of your back leg contracted.

YOU SHOULD FEEL IT

Working your glutes, hamstrings, quads, and stretching the hip flexor of your back leg.

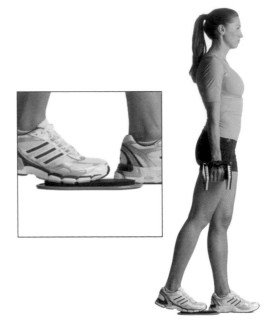

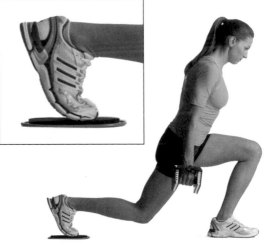

Romanian Deadlift (RDL) to Row—2 Arm, 1 Leg

STARTING POSITION

Stand on one foot facing a medium pulley cable station, holding the cable handles with both hands.

PROCEDURE

Keeping your down knee slightly bent and your back flat, hinge over at the hips and reach your arms out in front of you until you feel a mild stretch in your hamstrings. Return to standing position as you pull your elbows back and your forearms slide under your ribs. Continue for the prescribed number of reps and repeat on the other side.

COACHING KEY

Do not let your back round. Your torso and leg should move as one unit. Fire the glute of your extended leg to keep it straight. Keep your shoulder blades back and down throughout the movement. Keep the knee of your standing leg bent.

YOU SHOULD FEEL IT

In your glutes, hamstrings, and back.

Lateral Lunge to Drop Lunge—Slide

STARTING POSITION

Stand with your feet wider than shoulder-width apart, with your right foot on a slide, holding dumbbells atop your shoulder.

PROCEDURE

Slide your right foot laterally, keeping your leg straight and the bottom of your foot in contact with the slide. As you slide, squat back and down, keeping your weight on the left leg. Return to the starting position by

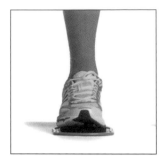

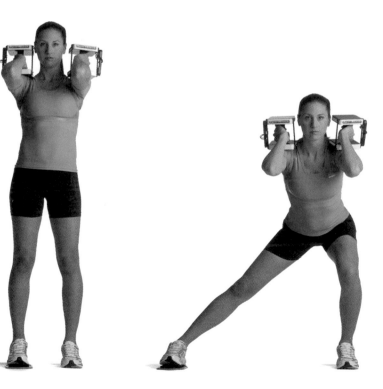

pushing up with the squatting leg. Next, reach your right foot 2 feet behind your left foot. Square your hips back to the starting position, and sit back and down into a squat. Return to the starting position and repeat for the prescribed number of reps, and switch sides.

COACHING KEY

Keep your toes pointed straight ahead and both feet in full contact with the ground and the slide.

YOU SHOULD FEEL IT

Working your glutes, hamstrings, and quads.

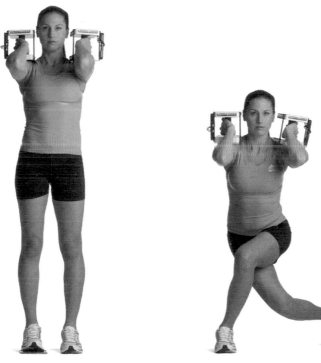

Romanian Deadlift (RDL) to Row— 1 Arm, 1 Leg

STARTING POSITION

Stand on your left foot facing a medium pulley cable station, holding the cable handles with your right hand.

PROCEDURE

Keeping your left knee slightly bent and your back flat, hinge over at the hips and reach your arm out in front of you until you feel a mild stretch in your hamstrings. Return to standing position as you pull your elbows back and your forearms slide under your ribs. Continue for the prescribed number of reps on each side.

COACHING KEY

Do not let your back round. Your torso and leg should move as one unit. Fire the glute of your extended leg to keep it straight. Keep your shoulder blades back and down throughout the movement. Keep your knee slightly bent.

YOU SHOULD FEEL IT

In your glutes, hamstrings, and back.

Romanian Deadlift (RDL) to Curl/Squat to Press

STARTING POSITION

Stand in an athletic position, feet, hip-width apart, with a pair of dumbbells at your sides.

PROCEDURE

Keeping your knees slightly bent, shift your hips back and lower the dumbbells as far as you can while keeping your back straight. As you stand up, curl the dumbbells to your shoulders. While holding them at your shoulders, squat your hips back and down. After you stand up, press the dumbbells over your head.

COACHING KEY

Fire your hamstrings and glutes as you return to an upright position. Don't think of the RDL exercise as bending forward; think of it as sitting back but with your torso moving forward instead of staying upright. Keep your knees slightly bent.

YOU SHOULD FEEL IT

In your glutes, hamstrings, quads, biceps, shoulders, and throughout your pillar.

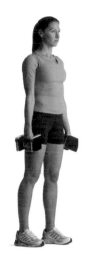
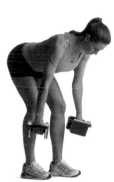
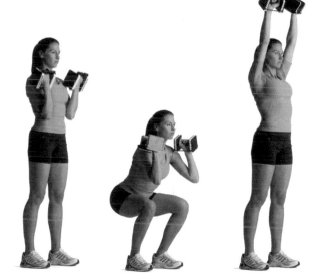

3-Hurdle Drill

STARTING POSITION

Lay three obstacles—towels, books, cups, or bricks, for example—each 2 to 3 feet apart from the next.

PROCEDURE

Begin by straddling the first obstacle. Run laterally over the obstacles, never crossing feet. Rapidly reverse direction.

COACHING KEY

Only your outside foot goes beyond the outside obstacles.

YOU SHOULD FEEL IT

Everywhere. This is a total-body exercise.

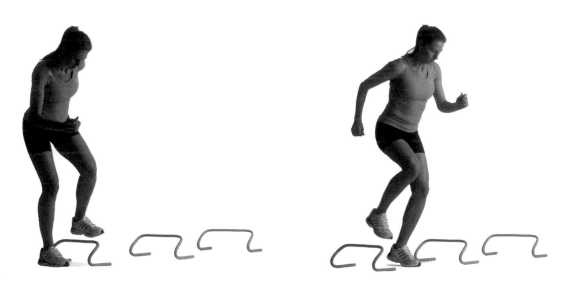

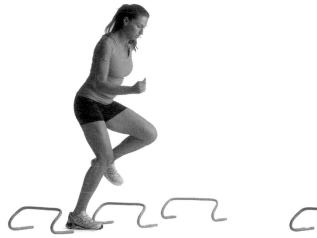
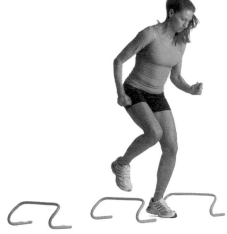
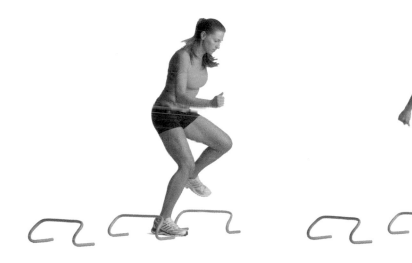

Squat Jump

STARTING POSITION

Stand with your feet just outside of your shoulders and your hands behind your head. Now sit back and down into a squat position, keeping your knees behind your toes.

PROCEDURE

After holding the starting position for 3 seconds, jump vertically. Pull your toes to your shins in midair to prepare for landing.

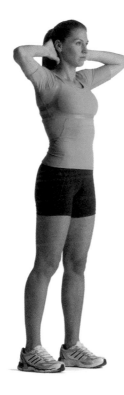
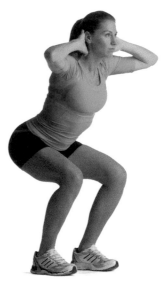

Land in the starting squat position, hold 3 seconds, and repeat for the prescribed number of times.

COACHING KEY

Keep your chest up during the jump and extend your hips completely. Land softly, with your hips back and down.

YOU SHOULD FEEL IT

Working your hips, knees, and ankles.

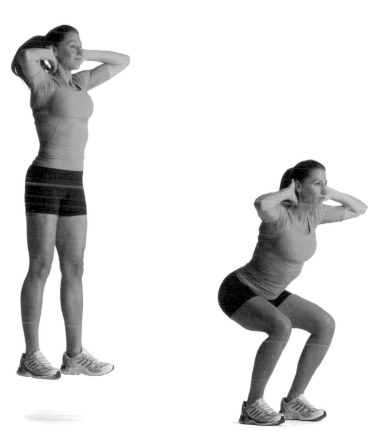

Burpee

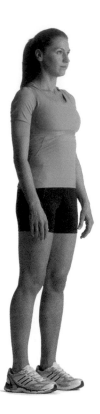

STARTING POSITION

Stand in an athletic position, with your feet outside your hips.

PROCEDURE

Squat down with your hands on the floor and jump out into a push-up position. Jump your feet back to your hands and then jump as high as you can with hands over your head.

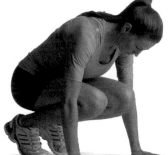

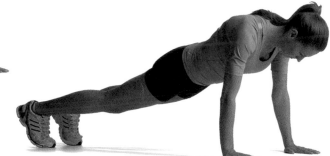

COACHING KEY

Land softly by sitting on your hips. Make sure your heels are on the ground when you finish the jump.

YOU SHOULD FEEL IT

Working your entire body and challenging your cardiovascular system.

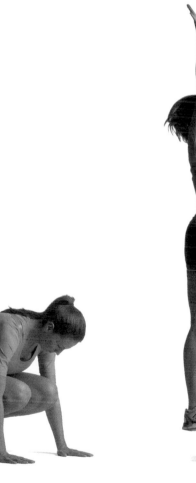

Rapid Response—2-Inch Runs

STARTING POSITION

Stand in an athletic position, with your feet outside your hips.

PROCEDURE

Keeping your toes pulled to the shin, run in place as fast as you can for the prescribed time. Contact with the ball of your foot. Your arms should move naturally and relaxed.

COACHING KEY

Keep your back flat and your toes pulled up to the shins. Don't scuff your feet on the ground; you should hear nice crisp pops as they strike the ground.

YOU SHOULD FEEL IT

Everywhere. This is a total-body exercise.

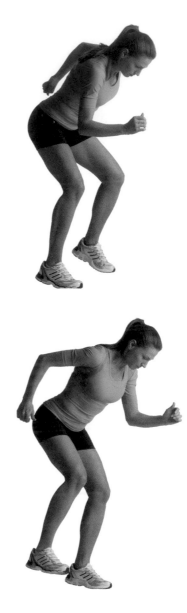

Bench Press—Alternating Dumbbell (with foam roll)

STARTING POSITION

Lie faceup on a foam roll placed along your spine, knees bent with your heels on the ground, your head resting at the top. Hold dumbbells at the edges of your shoulders, your palms facing your thighs.

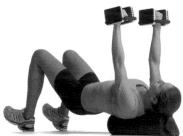

PROCEDURE

Lift both dumbbells straight up over your chest. Keeping one arm straight, lower the other dumbbell until your upper arm is parallel or slightly below parallel to the floor, then push it back up. Then repeat with the other arm. That's one repetition. Repeat for the prescribed number of reps.

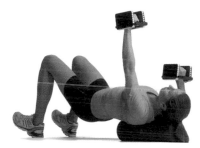

COACHING KEY

Make sure to stabilize your extended arm and take the active dumbbell through a full range of motion. Keep your stomach tight so your trunk does not rotate on the bench as the weight lowers.

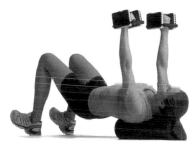

YOU SHOULD FEEL IT

In your chest, shoulders, and triceps.

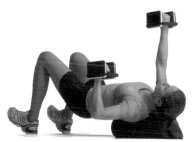

Bench Press—1-Arm Dumbbell (with foam roll)

STARTING POSITION

Lie faceup on a foam roll placed along your spine, knees bent with your heels on the ground, your head resting at the top.

PROCEDURE

Hold dumbbell in your left hand with your right arm straight out to your side, palm up. As you lower the weight with your left hand, keep the back of your right hand on the floor. Do all of the prescribed reps and switch sides.

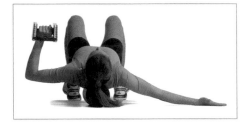

COACHING KEY

Keep your hips up throughout movement. Don't let anything move other than your arm.

YOU SHOULD FEEL IT

Working your torso, hips, and chest.

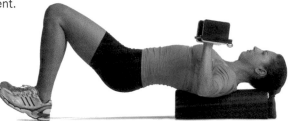

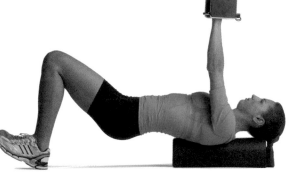

Push-up—Kneeling (Slides)

STARTING POSITION

Begin in a kneeling push-up position with your hands on slides.

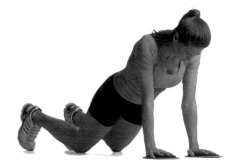

PROCEDURE

Start with your hands underneath your shoulders. As you lower into the load position, your hands slide apart. As you push up they slide back together. Repeat for the prescribed number of reps.

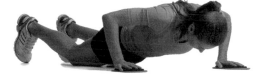

COACHING KEY

Keep your stomach tight throughout the movement and keep your knees, hips, and shoulders in line.

YOU SHOULD FEEL IT

Working your chest, shoulders, and torso.

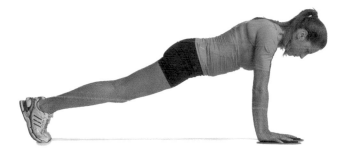

Glute Bridge to Hamstring Curl— Eccentric (Slides)

STARTING POSITION

Lie faceup on the floor, with both heels on slides.

PROCEDURE

Pull your heels toward your glutes. Lift your hips until your body is in a straight line from knee to shoulder. Keeping your hips extended and off the ground, slowly straighten your legs and then lower your hips to the ground. Repeat for the prescribed number of reps.

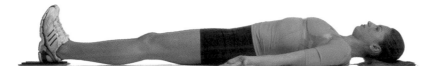

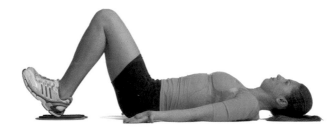

COACHING KEY

Do not let your hips drop as your heels move away from your glutes. Keep your toes pulled up.

YOU SHOULD FEEL IT

Working your glutes, hamstrings, and lower back.

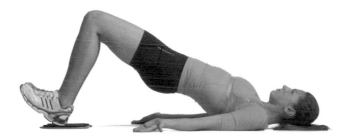

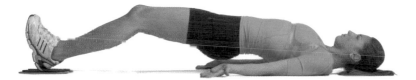

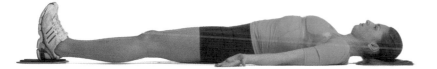

Glute Bridge to Hamstring Curl—Slides

STARTING POSITION

Lie faceup on the floor, knees bent, with both
heels on slides.

PROCEDURE

Fire the glutes and raise your hips so that
only your head, shoulders, arms, and feet are
touching the floor. Hold for the prescribed
amount of time.

COACHING KEY

Initiate the movement by firing the glutes and
keep them fired at the top of the movement.

YOU SHOULD FEEL IT

Strengthening and activating your
hamstrings, glutes, and lower back muscles.

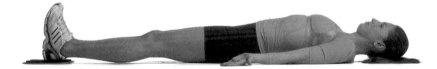

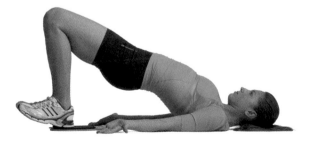

Chair Running

STARTING POSITION

Assume a push-up position with your hands on a chair or sofa. Your left knee is up to your chest as if in a sprinting position.

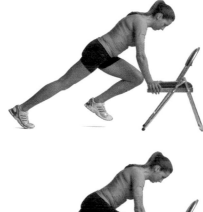

PROCEDURE

Run in place by switching legs in midair. If you start with your left knee to chest, like in a sprinter's acceleration position, switch in midair, keeping the movement continuous.

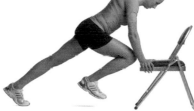

COACHING KEY

Don't let anything move in your torso— just your legs. Extend each leg fully with every rep.

YOU SHOULD FEEL IT

Working your torso, shoulders, and your cardiovascular system.

REGENERATION

Foam Roll—Thoracic Spine

STARTING POSITION

Lie faceup on the ground with your knees bent and heels on the ground with a foam roll under your midback and your head supported with your hands. Keep your elbows together.

PROCEDURE

Roll from the middle of your back up to your shoulders and repeat for 30 to 60 seconds.

COACHING KEY

Hold your hands behind your head with your elbows pointed to the sky and close together. Hold on sore sports for 30 to 60 seconds.

YOU SHOULD FEEL

As if you were getting a deep massage.

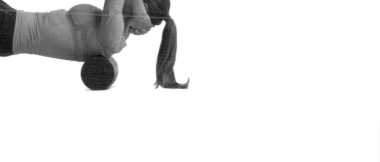

Thoracic Spine Mobility

STARTING POSITION

Tape two tennis balls together with athletic tape to form a peanut shape. Lie on your back, knees bent and heels on the ground with the balls under your spine just above your lower back and your hands behind your head.

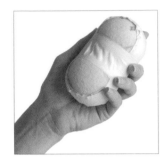

PROCEDURE

Perform 5 crunches, then raise your arms over your chest and alternately reach over your head for 5 repetitions with each arm. Move the balls up your spine for 1 to 2 inches and repeat the crunches and arm reaches. Continue moving the balls up your spine until they are just above your shoulder blades and below the base of your neck.

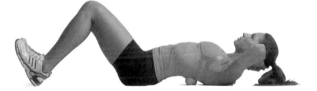

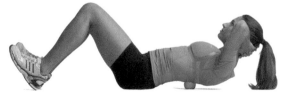

COACHING KEY

During the crunches, try to "hinge" on the ball rather than rolling over it. Think about keeping your ribs pushed down toward the ground during the arm reaches.

YOU SHOULD FEEL

As if you were getting a deep massage in your mid- to upper back.

Foam Roll—Calf

STARTING POSITION

Sit on the ground with your legs straight, your left leg crossed over the right, and a foam roll under your right calf.

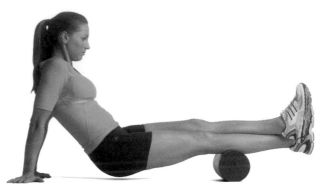

PROCEDURE

Lift your butt off the ground so that your weight is supported by your hands and the foam roll only. Roll the length of your calf, from your Achilles tendon to behind your knee, and repeat for 30 to 60 seconds per leg.

COACHING KEY

Place as much weight as possible on the roll. Hold on sore spots for 30 to 60 seconds.

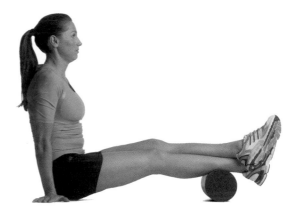

YOU SHOULD FEEL

As if you were getting a deep massage.

Foam Roll—Tibialis Anterior

STARTING POSITION

Get on your hands and knees with a foam roll under the front of your shins, just below your knees.

PROCEDURE

Keeping your hands still, roll your knees toward your hands, rolling the front of your shins from just below your knees to your ankles. Repeat for 30 to 60 seconds.

COACHING KEY

Keep your back flat and stomach tight throughout the movement. Place as much weight as possible on the roll. Hold on sore spots for 30 to 60 seconds.

YOU SHOULD FEEL

As if you were getting a deep massage.

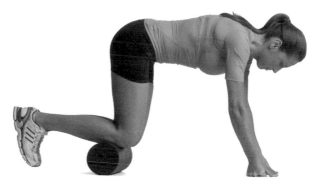

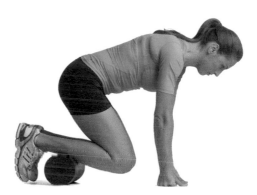

Foam Roll—Hamstring

STARTING POSITION
Sit on the ground with a foam roll under the back of one thigh and the other leg crossed over it.

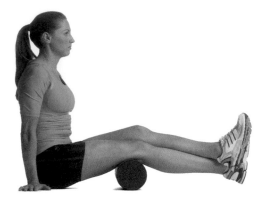

PROCEDURE
Roll up and down the length of the back of your thigh, for 30 to 60 seconds. Then switch legs and repeat.

COACHING KEY
If the massage feels too sensitive, uncross your legs and roll both hamstrings at once. Hold on sore spots for 30 to 60 seconds.

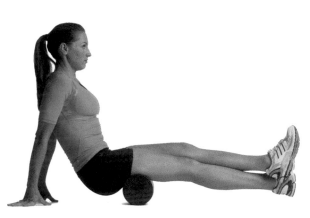

YOU SHOULD FEEL
As if you were getting a deep massage.

Foam Roll—Quad/Hip Flexor

STARTING POSITION

Lie facedown on the ground, supported on your elbows, with a foam roll under one thigh and the other leg crossed at the ankles.

PROCEDURE

Roll along the quads from your hip to just above your knees for 30 to 60 seconds, then repeat on the other side.

COACHING KEY

For added benefit, roll slightly on the outside and inside as well as down the front of the thigh. Hold on sore spots for 30 to 60 seconds.

YOU SHOULD FEEL

As if you were getting a deep massage.

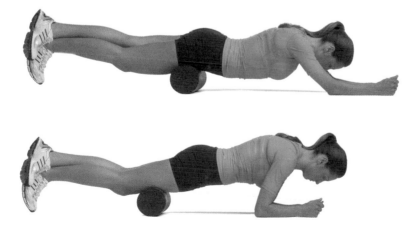

Foam Roll—IT (Iliotibial) Band

STARTING POSITION

Lie on your side with a foam roll under the outside of your thigh.

PROCEDURE

Roll over the foam from your hip to just above your knee, then repeat on the other side.

COACHING KEY

Hold on sore spots for 30 to 60 seconds.

YOU SHOULD FEEL

As if you were getting a deep massage.

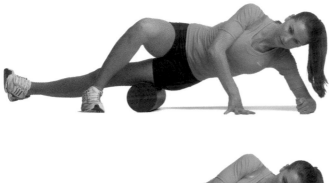

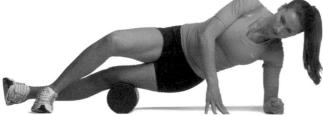

Foam Roll—TFL (Tensor Fasciae Latae)

STARTING POSITION

Lie facedown, supported on your elbows, with
a foam roll under your hip.

PROCEDURE

Roll along the muscle on the front and
slightly to the outside of your upper thigh
just below the pelvis for 30 to 60 seconds
per leg.

COACHING KEY

Hold on sore spots for 30 to 60 seconds.

YOU SHOULD FEEL

As if you were getting a deep massage.

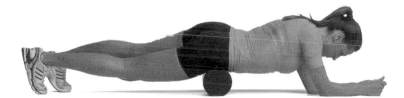

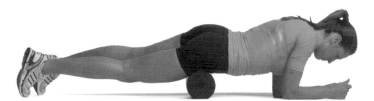

Foam Roll—Glute

STARTING POSITION

Sit on the ground with a foam roll slightly below your buttocks.

PROCEDURE

Roll along the length of your glute for 30 to 60 seconds.

COACHING KEY

Hold on sore spots for 30 to 60 seconds.

YOU SHOULD FEEL

As if you were getting a deep massage.

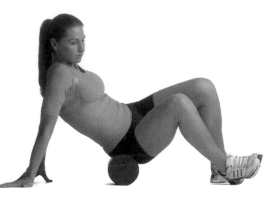

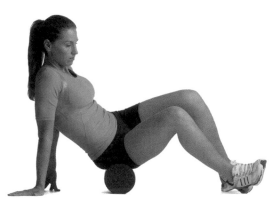

Foam Roll—Lower Back and QL
(Quadratus Lumborum)

STARTING POSITION

Lie faceup on the ground with a foam roll
under the outside of your midback, just below
your rib cage.

PROCEDURE

Roll from the middle of your back down to
your pelvis and repeat for 30 to 60 seconds.

COACHING KEY

Hold on sore spots for 30 to 60 seconds.

YOU SHOULD FEEL

As if you were getting a deep massage.

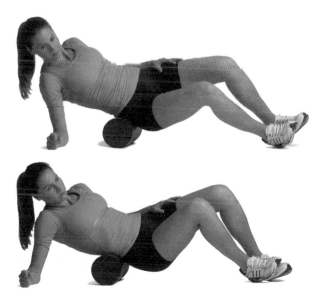

Foam Roll—Chest

STARTING POSITION

Lie facedown on the ground with one arm extended, a foam roll placed under the armpit of the extended arm.

PROCEDURE

Roll under the arm and over that side of the chest for 30 to 60 seconds. Then switch arms and repeat.

COACHING KEY

Hold on sore spots for 30 to 60 seconds.

YOU SHOULD FEEL

As if you were getting a deep massage.

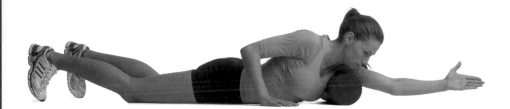

FLEXIBILITY EXERCISES

The following flexibility exercises will help bring balance back to your body. Active-isolated stretching will help lengthen short or stiff muscles by reprogramming your muscles to contract and relax through new ranges of motion. These exercises will help relieve tension throughout your body and alleviate the associated aches and pains. Hold each stretch for 2 seconds while exhaling, then relax and continue for 10 repetitions each.

Reach, Roll—Foam Roll

STARTING POSITION

Sit on your heels with your arms extended
and the backs of your hands on a foam roll.

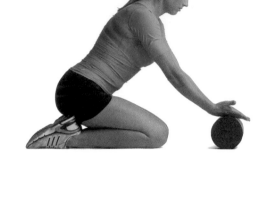

PROCEDURE

Roll the foam forward while keeping your hips
back and your chest dropped toward the
ground. Exhale as you hold the stretch for 2
seconds. Return to the starting position and
repeat.

COACHING KEY

Attempt to lift your hands off
the foam roll as you exhale,
but keep your hands in
contact with the foam.

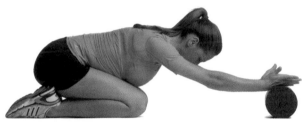

YOU SHOULD FEEL

Stretching in your upper back
and shoulders.

AIS Bent-Knee Hamstring

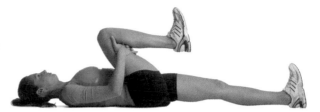

STARTING POSITION

Lie on your back with both legs straight. Pull your right knee to your chest, grasping behind the knee with both hands.

PROCEDURE

Actively straighten your right knee as much as possible without letting it move away from your chest. Hold 2 seconds, and relax. Continue for 10 repetitions, then switch legs and repeat.

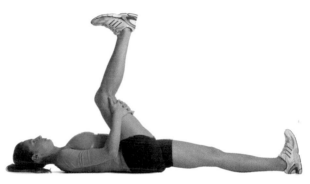

COACHING KEY

Keep your opposite leg on the ground by pushing your heel as far away from your head as possible, contracting your glute. Keep your knee pulled as tightly to your chest as possible throughout the entire movement. It's okay if you can't fully straighten your knee.

YOU SHOULD FEEL

Stretching in the hamstring of the bent leg and stretching in the hip flexor of the bottom leg.

AIS Kneeling Quad/Hip Flexor

STARTING POSITION
Half kneel (put one knee on the ground) with your back knee on a soft mat or pad. Rest your hands on your forward knee.

PROCEDURE
While keeping a slight forward lean in your torso, tighten your stomach and contract the glute of your back leg. Maintaining this posture, shift your entire body slightly forward. Exhale and hold the stretch for 2 seconds. Relax, repeat 10 times, and then switch legs.

COACHING KEY
Avoid excessive arching in your lower back.

YOU SHOULD FEEL
Stretching in the front of your hip and upper thigh of your back leg.

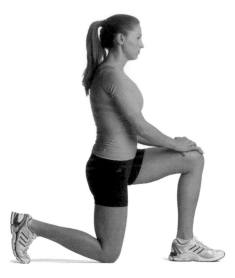

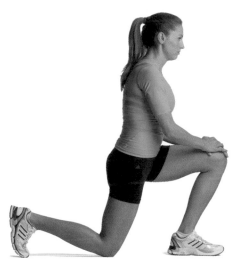

AIS Abductor

STARTING POSITION

Lie on your back with both legs straight.

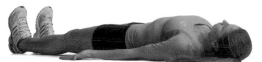

PROCEDURE

Lift your right knee to your chest, placing your right hand on your knee and your left hand under your ankle. Pull your right leg as close as you can to your chest into a gentle stretch while contracting your left glute. Hold the stretch for 2 seconds, and then relax. Continue for 10 repetitions, then switch legs and repeat.

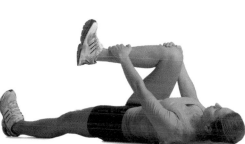

COACHING KEY

Throughout the movement, contract the glute of the leg that's on the ground, point that foot toward the ceiling, and keep your belly button drawn in.

YOU SHOULD FEEL

Stretching in the outside of the hip of your bent leg.

AIS Kneeling Adductor

STARTING POSITION

Half kneel (put one knee on the ground) with your back knee on a soft mat or pad. Rest your hands on your forward knee.

PROCEDURE

With your front foot pointed toward 10 o'clock or 2 o'clock, depending on the leg, slide your hips toward your front foot until you feel a stretch on the inside of your thigh. Hold for 1 to 2 seconds, then relax. Continue for 10 repetitions, then switch legs and repeat.

COACHING KEY

Don't let your back foot rotate during the movement.

YOU SHOULD FEEL IT

Stretching the inside of your thigh on your back leg.

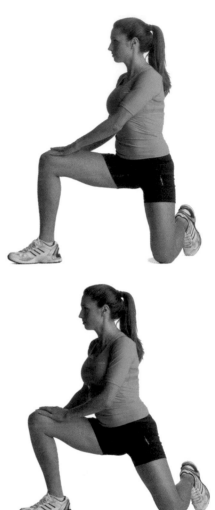

AIS Side-Lying Shoulder Stretch

STARTING POSITION

Lie on your side with the upper part of your bottom arm parallel to your belt line and your top elbow bent 90 degrees.

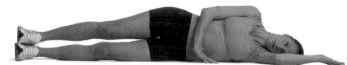

PROCEDURE

Rotate the palm of your bottom hand toward the ground as far as possible, gently pressing your palm farther with the other hand. Hold for 2 seconds, relax, and repeat 10 times. Then switch sides.

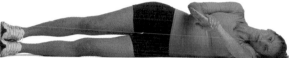

COACHING KEY

Actively try to rotate your palm toward the ground throughout the entire movement. Keep your chin tucked and do not let your bottom shoulder rise off the ground. Start with a small range of motion and gradually increase it.

YOU SHOULD FEEL

Stretching in your back and the inside of your bottom shoulder.

TRIGGER POINT EXERCISES

Trigger point exercises will work similarly to the foam roll; however, with the following exercises it will be much easier to isolate and release deeper tissues. Each one should feel as if you were getting a deep massage. Spend 30 to 60 seconds on each muscle, holding on any sore spots you find for an additional 30 to 60 seconds to release the tissue.

Trigger Point—Arch

STARTING POSITION

Stand with your shoes off.

PROCEDURE

Place one foot on a golf ball or tennis ball. Roll the arch of your foot back and forth over the ball 50 times. Hold on any trigger point for 30 to 90 seconds. Then switch feet and repeat.

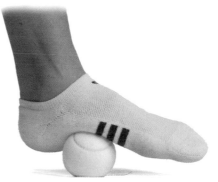

COACHING KEY

The more uncomfortable it is, the more your muscle needs to be massaged. Hold on sore spots for an extended time to release them. Roll through different angles to cover the entire arch of your foot.

YOU SHOULD FEEL

As if you were getting a deep massage on the bottom of your foot.

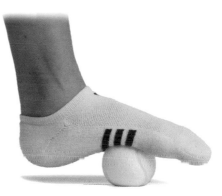

Trigger Point—VMO
(Vastus Medialis Obliquus)

STARTING POSITION

Lie on your stomach with a tennis ball just above your knee.

PROCEDURE

Adjust your position on the ball until you find a sore trigger point. Hold on the spot for 60 to 90 seconds. Repeat on the other side.

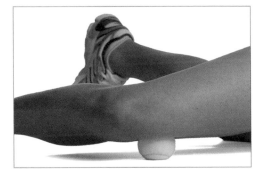

COACHING KEY

Try to maintain as much body weight on the ball as possible. The more uncomfortable it is, the more your muscle needs to be massaged.

YOU SHOULD FEEL

As if you were getting a deep massage on your VMO.

Trigger Point—TFL (Tensor Fasciae Latae)

STARTING POSITION

Lie facedown, supported on your elbows, with a tennis ball under one hip.

PROCEDURE

Roll on the front and slightly to the outside of your upper thigh just below the pelvis for 30 to 60 seconds. Switch legs and repeat.

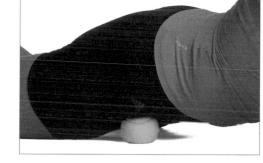

COACHING KEY

Try to maintain as much body weight on the ball as possible. The more uncomfortable it is, the more your muscle needs to be massaged. Hold on sore spots for 30 to 60 seconds.

YOU SHOULD FEEL

As if you were getting a deep massage.

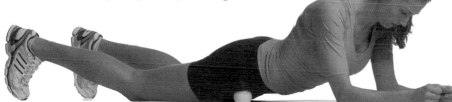

Trigger Point—Glute

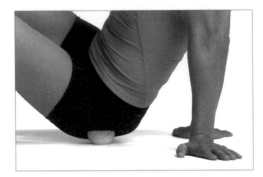

STARTING POSITION

Sit on one hip with a tennis ball under the outside of one of your glutes.

PROCEDURE

Adjust your position on the ball until you find a sore trigger point. Hold on the spot for 60 to 90 seconds. Move the ball to a slightly different spot and repeat. Repeat on the other side.

COACHING KEY

Try to maintain as much body weight on the ball as possible. The more uncomfortable it is, the more your muscle needs to be massaged. If you experience numbness or tingling in your foot, adjust the ball to a different spot.

YOU SHOULD FEEL

As if you were getting a deep massage to your glute and piriformis (a muscle in your hip rotator complex).

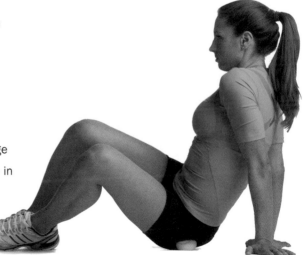

Trigger Point—Neck

STARTING POSITION

Lie on your back with two tennis balls taped together placed just below your neck.

PROCEDURE

Adjust your position on the balls until you find a sore trigger point. Hold on the spot for 60 to 90 seconds.

COACHING KEY

Try to maintain as much body weight on the balls as possible. The more uncomfortable it is, the more your muscle needs to be massaged.

YOU SHOULD FEEL

As if you were getting a deep massage in your neck.

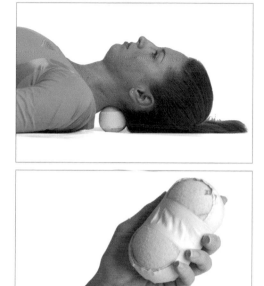

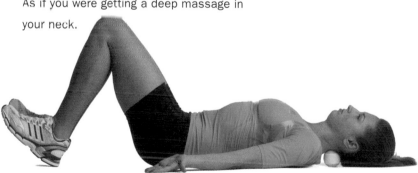

Trigger Point—Posterior Shoulder

STARTING POSITION

Lie on your side with the upper part of
your bottom arm parallel to your belt line
and your top elbow bent 90 degrees, a
tennis ball under your shoulder.

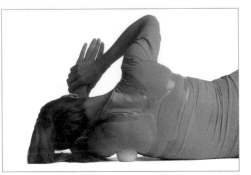

PROCEDURE

Adjust your position on the ball until you
find a sore trigger point. Hold on the
spot for 60 to 90 seconds. Repeat on
the other side.

COACHING KEY

Try to maintain as much body weight on
the ball as possible. The more
uncomfortable it is, the more your
muscle needs to be massaged.

YOU SHOULD FEEL

As if you were getting a deep massage in
your shoulder.

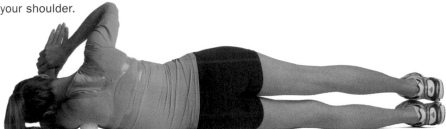

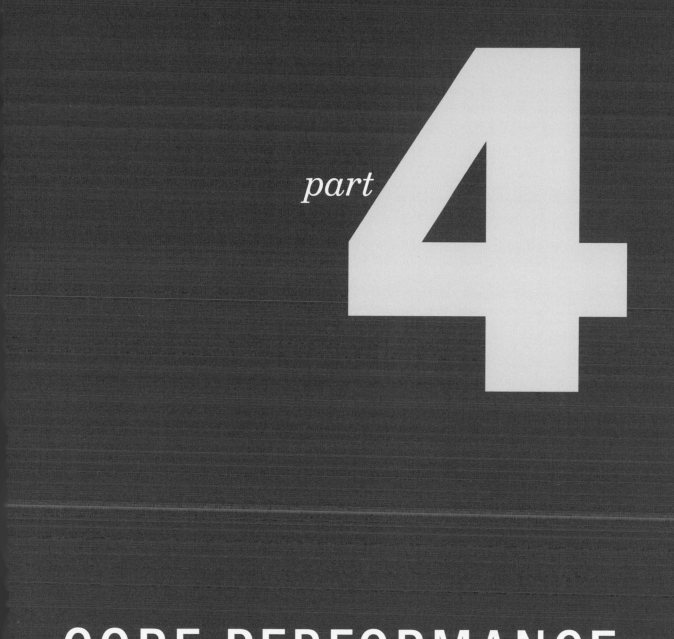

part *4*

CORE PERFORMANCE
RECOVERY

CHAPTER

12

REGENERATION

There's a tendency to think recovery, or what I call Regeneration, does not matter. At the very least, some people—even some of the top names in sports—presume they don't need any help in this area.

After all, everyone knows how to rest and recover. That's the easy part, right?

Why, I'm an expert at lying on the couch watching television or sitting by the pool reading a book. Yes, give me enough time and I'll show you some world-class resting and relaxation!

Notice the key phrase in that statement. Give me enough time. I'm always amazed at how many women (and men) cannot name the last vacation they took. I like to read those at-a-glance bio boxes of successful businesspeople that appear in magazine articles. They'll list the ages of their kids, favorite movies, what's currently on their iPod, and so on. Inevitably they'll be asked about their most recent vacation.

"Long weekend at the beach . . . two years ago."

Amazing, isn't it? These usually are people with the financial resources to take exotic vacations that most people never could experience. Yet they opt not to in part because they subscribe to this misguided belief that getting more done means working longer and longer.

At some point in the last decade it became fashionable, even a point of pride, not to take any vacation. It used to be you'd brag about your vacation, subject friends to looking at dozens of photos, and start planning your next journey the moment you got home.

These days people are reachable via cell phone and e-mail all the time. Many work from home or wherever they happen to be. We've blurred the lines between work and rest. Everyone, it seems, is working all the time. Nobody has time for anything. Instead of bragging about vacations, we talk about how "slammed" we are.

Being busy is the modern-day status symbol, even if it's being busy with unpleasant things.

Admittedly, when the economy is suffering, those of us still working are thankful to be in such a position. It's also true that some of those folks I read about in magazines are entrepreneurs flying by the seat of their pants in the early stages of building their companies, without the luxury of taking a vacation.

But there's another group, the vast majority I'd say, who have simply forgotten how to relax. The sad thing is that they're costing themselves not only the wonderful opportunities for personal and family growth that vacation provides, but they're also compromising the very productivity and earning power they so treasure.

If you're working hard all the time, you're never truly recovered. You might be working hard, but you're not working smart. On the contrary—you're so mentally and physically fatigued that you're not nearly as productive as you think you are.

Regeneration—or "Regen"—is not just a physical philosophy. The time spent at rest is when we enjoy the fruits of our labor. Not only that, but we also recharge our batteries and come back invigorated and stronger, ready to perform at even higher levels.

Regeneration, quite simply, is a lifestyle philosophy, a recognition that you need to plan ways to recover—mentally and physically—in all areas of your life. You actually experience the benefit of your hard work on the days that you rest.

This applies to your workout and your life. After you work out and eat properly, your body experiences the benefit—and grows—while you're at rest and even sleeping. Likewise you enjoy the benefits of your long weeks and months of work when you take that amazing vacation, whether you do so alone or are able to share the experience with others.

Otherwise what would be the point of all of that hard work? That's why Regeneration is an equal fourth pillar of the Core Performance Women system, along with Mindset, Nutrition, and Movement. Regeneration can—and should—be the most enjoyable part of the program if you just remember this simple formula:

Work + Rest = Success

Regeneration also is something you must work into every day, week, month, and year. At the moment do you actively work recovery into your daily schedule? Into your yearly schedule? Do you actively work recovery into your weekly exercise plan? Do you understand the effective methods to recover, and do you allow your body to constantly regenerate to meet the demands of life?

We take less vacation in the United States than most countries on the planet. Four to six weeks of vacation are commonplace in Europe, and that does not seem to have cost them any productivity. You might not agree with the practical aspects of that system, but I'd be willing to bet it improves productivity, since it allows Europeans to recharge their batteries, reconnect with families, and enjoy some of the best vacation destinations in the world.

If you do nothing else with this program, I hope you schedule regular vacations. That's the first thing I do when I lay out my calendar for the upcoming year. I block out my vacations in ink. If I don't, someone else is going to claim that time.

Regeneration isn't just about serving as your own travel agent. It's about recovering from the stresses of everyday life, as well as from the rigors of this program.

Remember, this program will only be moderately successful if you have a limiting lifestyle, and for many women that limitation comes in the form of a lack of sleep. Sleep is a vital component of regeneration. It rebuilds our bodies, releases rejuvenating hormones, and allows us to stay alert throughout the day, hitting the brain's "refresh" button.

In 2001 the National Sleep Foundation performed its famous "Sleep in America" survey, determining that 63 percent of adults get less than the recommended eight hours of sleep per night and 31 percent get less than seven hours. More than 40 percent of adult Americans reported having trouble staying awake during the day.

Sleep deprivation can interfere with memory, energy levels, mental ability, and mood. Without sleep you simply cannot function at your best. Sleep debt undermines your ability to eat healthfully and exercise as well, thus raising your level of body fat. When the brain is exhausted, it doesn't know whether it is sleep-deprived or starving for glucose, so the natural response is to crave sugar, which is why you have late-night cravings when you're tired. When you're low on energy, your brain wants to conserve energy, so motivation to exercise is greatly reduced.

Not getting enough sleep is harmful enough, but it's often combined with late-night eating and alcohol consumption. Even if you don't drink excessively, a couple of beers or cocktails inhibit sleep and contribute to weight gain.

Earlier we discussed the health benefits of *moderate* consumption of red wine. But remember also that it's difficult to reap the rewards of this program if recreational drinking is a key part of your lifestyle. (It goes without saying that smoking is counterproductive to healthy living.)

Sleep, though, is the most underrated aspect of a healthy lifestyle. For all the talk of improving nutrition and exercise, we tend to ignore this obvious lifestyle component. As kindergarteners we learn the restorative powers of a nap, placing our heads on our desks. Unfortunately we quickly break this powerful habit. An afternoon siesta of just twenty to thirty minutes can give you a second wind for the rest of the day.

Our approach to recovery and regeneration starts with a commitment to build recovery into every day, week, month, and year. Look for opportunities to allot time for relaxation, whether at work or at home, even if it's only fifteen minutes. Focus on self-regenerative techniques such as self-massage, flexibility exercises, and hydrotherapy (such as hot and cold contrasts). This approach should also hold true in your weekly plan, where you're planning a morning or an evening off or some activity that allows you to psychologically and physically recover, like going for a walk, enjoying a hot tub or bath, or scheduling a massage. More broadly, apply the same concept to each month and, ultimately, by building in proactive vacations or breaks to each quarter of the year or to the holiday breaks.

The specific strategies we'll discuss in this chapter help reset your muscle length to protect your long-term posture. These routines decrease the potential for pain and will jump-start your recovery.

Regeneration starts with how we plan our training. We'll schedule regeneration into each day, and we'll schedule regeneration days during the course of the week. In addition to keeping a regeneration mindset and doing specific Regen workouts to improve the quality of your tissue, you'll see the concept of regeneration built into the nutrition program as well.

Think of regeneration in terms of *active* regeneration and *passive* regeneration.

Active regeneration consists of easy aerobic activity, such as a bike ride, run, or short segment on a piece of exercise equipment. The idea here is to avoid pounding and huge energy expenditure but still do something for circulation and to help move nutrients in and out of the cells.

Passive regeneration involves such activities as massages and hot and cold contrasts (more on those in a minute). But passive regeneration is also a mindset, the idea that we're working constantly to become better, even when we're not working out. This philosophy includes getting proper sleep—even taking naps—and planning ahead to make the most of time. It also involves taking vacations and enjoying leisure pursuits.

The regeneration unit requires some inexpensive items: a massage stick, foam roll, stretch rope, and massage/pressure point ball. Each one of them will help you iron out the muscles and also help you maintain great posture. These simple devices can be tossed in your gym bag or can occupy a small area of your home. Some of our athletes have found it convenient to place the items in a small basket at the side of a couch, easily accessible when relaxing or watching TV at night.

Our goal with regeneration is not to do *more*, but to integrate these routines into the relaxation periods you have scheduled in your normal daily routines. I believe that once you try them and experience them, you will look forward to reinvesting in and reinvigorating yourself at the end of your workday.

Self-Massage

Tissue is like a rubber band. Our goal is to keep it supple and elastic. Unfortunately it tends to get knotted up with spasms over time. If you put twenty knots into a rubber band, it's the same rubber band, but it doesn't store nearly as much energy. More stress goes into a few parts of the rubber band instead of dispersing throughout the band. The goal with our self-massage is to undo the knots and spasms. Once we get those worked out, we need to address them daily and weekly to make sure that no more knots accumulate. It takes consistent, proactive maintenance.

The foam roll is an eighteen-inch-long roll of tightly packed foam, roughly five inches in diameter. You rotate and roll your hamstrings, quadriceps, back, lats, and hips over the foam roll to release the spasms and accelerate your body's recovery.

This works because the foam roll routine is like a massage. It uses deep compression to help roll out the muscle spasms that develop over time. The compression overstimulates the nerves, which signal the muscle spasm to shut off. This allows the muscles to relax and loosen up, gets the blood and lymphatic system flowing, and helps reestablish a healthy muscle and body. Think of your body as clay. The roll softens up the clay, so you can remold it into something more pliable and functional.

You'll probably enjoy the foam-roll routine—everyone likes massages. Still, there will be some uncomfortable moments, as there are with a professional massage. Once you're past the first few weeks, though, it will become considerably easier and more comfortable. The foam roll is a great barometer of the quality of your muscle and connective tissue. The better it feels, and the less it hurts, the higher the quality of your tissue.

As you roll on the foam, discovering muscle spasms and pressure points, you'll knead out the knots by working in a small pattern back and forth for thirty seconds and then holding on that pressure point for an additional thirty to sixty seconds until the muscle cries mercy and releases from spasm. This process will continue to iron out the muscles throughout the course of the week.

Our versatile massage stick, available at www.coreperformance.com—is a simple yet revolutionary device that compresses and stretches muscle. Made of plastic beads, it provides an effective self-massage that may be done before, during, or after a workout. The massage stick releases muscle spasms while increasing blood and lymphatic flow in the body. In addition, we've added small eyelets on each end of the device that enable you to use the stick for the stability lifting, chopping, and rotation exercises that progress from this program. Thus we're able to "lengthen then strengthen" our bodies for these specific movements.

Flexibility Exercises

Self-massage helps untangle the knots, but you also must build flexibility, an integral component of the Core Performance Women program. From Movement Prep to nearly every exercise, flexibility is key to achieving your fitness goals. Active-isolated stretching (AIS), developed by Aaron Mattes to target specific muscles that get short or stiff from the demands of life, will help you dramatically improve your flexibility. (You can learn more about it at www.coreperformance.com.)

The key to AIS is its *active* nature. To perform the stretches, you won't stretch for ten to thirty seconds, as in traditional stretching

Instead you'll hold each stretch for just one to two seconds, thus increasing the muscles' range of motion a few more degrees with each repetition. Exhale during the hold position, releasing tension and getting a deeper stretch. Return to the starting position and repeat for the desired number of reps. With this type of exercise you have to put your "mind in the muscle" to focus on firing the proper muscles and relaxing the muscles to be stretched.

More than working your muscles, you're reprogramming your brain. As an example, the hamstring stretch requires you to lie on your back, with your hands behind a knee, pulling the knee to your chest. As you extend your knee, those muscles contract, and your hamstrings automatically relax, through a process called reciprocal inhibition. Hold that position for a two-second count as you exhale and release the tension from your body and mind. Two seconds might not seem like much, especially if you're used to static stretching routines, but this is a gradual process that will yield a few degrees with each repetition over the course of eight to ten reps, ultimately resulting in significant increases in flexibility.

You also can do AIS exercises using an eight- to ten-foot length of rope, about the thickness of a jump rope. You can go to a home improvement store and have a length cut off for just a few dollars, or you can check out the ropes at www.coreperformance .com, which come with an instructional DVD.

If you wrap the rope around one foot at a time and perform a series of moves, you will reprogram your muscles to contract and relax through new ranges of motion. For a hamstring stretch, you lie on your back with a rope wrapped around one leg. Lift your leg as far as you can into the air, then pull your toe up toward your shin, then squeeze, or "fire," your quadriceps, hip flexors, and abs. Give gentle assistance by pulling on the rope and then holding for two seconds. Return to the starting position and continue for eight to ten repetitions.

You should also use traditional static stretching post-workout. Here we'll hold for thirty seconds to three minutes to improve long-term structural flexibility. You can learn other great stretching techniques from a talented woman named Ann Frederick at www.stretchtowin.com.

However, as a rule of thumb, avoid static stretching prior to working out—static stretching works by putting the muscle and the nervous system in a submissive hold until it shuts off and releases. The last thing you want to do is have your muscles shut off prior to using them. As a general rule, static stretching should be limited to post-workout and days off.

Contrasts

At Athletes' Performance, athletes alternate between sitting for three to five minutes in a hot tub followed by one minute to three minutes in a 55-degree "cold plunge" tub. The cold therapy in particular decreases the natural post-workout muscle inflammation and can be used alone for six to ten minutes immediately after a workout.

When you enter the warm water, the blood flows out to your skin and limbs to in-

CORE WOMEN SUCCESS STORY

"I could mold and shape my body."

Trish Kinney • Age: Fifty-six • Hometown: Tempe, Arizona

In 1995 Trish Kinney underwent surgery at the Mayo Clinic to remove a large, malignant breast mass along with forty lymph nodes, eighteen of which were infected with cancer.

She underwent an unusual type of bone marrow transplant, known as a stem cell rescue, spending a month in a sterile room making a new immune system from her own donated stem cells. She left the hospital worn out and without hair, but emotionally and spiritually energized.

After a successful recovery, further challenges were in store. Chemotherapy had led to "instant" menopause at the age of forty-three. A lifelong dancer, she always had enjoyed a lean, lithe body. Seemingly overnight she gained eleven pounds and watched her waist disappear. Worst of all, her bones began a downward spiral into full-blown osteoporosis.

"I realized I had earned a new life, but I wasn't prepared for this new body," she says. "It was a huge setback emotionally. I felt like a stranger in my own skin."

Kinney gave up dancing, her greatest joy. She simply couldn't bear going into the studio looking the way she did. For the first time in her life she changed her diet and began working out every day. But because she had so little expertise in anything but dance, the results were not what she hoped for.

"I worked hard but knew I wasn't meeting my physical potential and was unhappy with the way I looked and felt," she says. "After struggling for a long while, I maintained a more acceptable weight but was still unsatisfied."

A longtime Tempe resident, Kinney read about Mark Verstegen's Athletes' Performance training center and inquired about its executive program. Soon she was following a regimen similar to those used by Verstegen's pro athletes.

Having retained good mobility and flexibility from dancing, Kinney was surprised and delighted to discover how much of the program incorporated movement and stretching, which felt familiar and comfortable. And she was enthused about the strength training that was less familiar but results driven. She began to recapture the body she remembered, only stronger.

One afternoon she watched a baseball pitcher who was rehabilitating an injured shoulder execute his windup and delivery during a throwing session. She marveled at the aesthetics of the movement and realized that she was gradually regaining her own movement patterns, through her own rehab from serious illness and its physical challenges.

"I learned that I could mold and shape my body using the combination of nutrition and training taught through Core Performance. I felt I could be just as exceptional in my own way as pro athletes using the same methods. I knew I wouldn't have the same body I did at age twenty-five or thirty, but I did want a mature, recognizable version of it. Even as a middle-aged woman with body issues, this program made it possible. It was everything I was looking for, a guide to success."

Finally she was ready to go back into the dance studio. The mirrors reflected her fit, limber body and the movement came naturally.

Gradually she noticed that she was incorporating dance into her everyday life again, gliding across the hardwood floors of her big kitchen while cooking dinner.

"I don't need an audience anymore. I dance for myself, for the pure joy of it. I have a body now that tells me for the first time in years that I am actually dancing again."

A year after starting the Core Performance program, Kinney's body fat percentage and lean muscle mass improved significantly. Her annual tests at Mayo Clinic showed that not only had her bone loss stabilized, but she had achieved a 6 percent improvement in bone density, no longer at osteoporosis level. Doctors dubbed her "Iron Woman."

She prefers "The Incredible Hulk" nickname she earned at Athletes' Performance for adding lean mass to her small dancer's frame. It is a title she wears proudly, knowing her new-found strength is vital going forward.

"I will always be in a lifelong battle against this disease," she says. "I don't have it anymore but the war is waged every single day. Core Performance has prepared me for that battle. It is life-changing."

crease the surface area through which heat can dissipate—just as your skin flushes when exercising in the heat. The cold does the opposite, pulling blood away from the skin and limbs and toward the heart, not unlike what happens when your fingers turn blue in extreme cold. After a workout this contrast stimulates muscle recovery with little effort.

Hot and cold contrasts force your blood to move fast, from deep in your trunk out to your limbs and skin and then back again. That's a good thing in and of itself. But when you do it immediately after a workout and on Regeneration days, you stimulate blood flow and muscle recovery with hardly any effort. (Resistance training and ESD requires energy and creates tiny micro-tears in muscle fibers, which your body repairs in between workouts, leaving your muscles ready to adapt to further training.) You don't need access to a hot tub or a cold plunge; you can get the same effect in the shower by switching between hot and cold settings. If you want to end your contrasts feeling fresh and energized, end on the cold setting. If you're looking to wind down at the end of the day, finish hot.

CHAPTER 12 SUMMARY: Regeneration is a recognition that you need to plan ways to recover in all areas of your life. That way you'll experience the benefit of work on the days you rest. (Remember: Work + Rest = Success.) The time spent at rest is when we clear our minds and enjoy the fruits of our labor, when we realize the gains produced by all of our hard work. Not only that, we also recharge our batteries and come back invigorated and stronger, ready to perform at even higher levels. These measures include proper planning, nutrition, sleep, active-isolated and static stretching, foam roll work, and hot and cold contrasts.

AFTERWORD:
KEEPING SCORE

My favorite part about writing books is the feedback I receive from people who have used the Core Performance system to overcome pain, lose weight, increase flexibility, and initiate a plan for high-performance movement and nutrition for long-term health and success.

I've literally been brought from goose bumps to tears by some of the e-mails and letters I've received from folks who have benefited from this program, and I am deeply honored to have helped put them on the path to success. Some of these women you've already read about in these pages. I hope to hear from you as well, if not soon then perhaps years from now.

That's because the Core Performance system will sustain you for the rest of your life. This program is an ongoing process and we offer you progressions and variations on these workouts here and online that can support you indefinitely. You'll notice we did not present this as a "6-Week Plan for Success" or "12 Weeks to a Better You." The idea is not to get in the best shape or your life for some short-term goal but rather to develop a long-term, sustainable system that will power your performance forever.

Core Performance is not just a workout routine. By picking up this book, you have entered into the Core Performance community, which allows you to benefit from the "Core Values and Fundamentals to Perform in the Game of Life." Books are a terrific medium to share thoughts and ideas to help readers improve the quality of their lives, and that's been the goal of *Core Performance Women*.

For additional information, you might check out one of our previous four books, all available in paperback. If you enjoy golf, you might be especially interested in the book *Core Performance Golf*, which will put yards on your drive and take strokes off your score. If you're someone passionate about running, swimming, cycling, or triathlon, *Core Performance Endurance* will lower your times and show you how to train more efficiently. Our first two books, *Core Performance* and *Core Performance Essentials*, introduced the program to hundreds of thousands of readers and remain timeless resources.

Many of our readers have found it useful to watch DVDs of our workouts as a reminder and a useful aid in performing these exercises properly. We have specific DVD products for golf and other sports, along with the general Core Performance system, available at our Web site, www.coreperformance.com, as well as at retail stores such as Target, Dick's Sporting Goods, and most other national specialty chains via our industry-leading partner, GoFit.

We hope you'll continue to reference this book for many years to come. At the same time, we want to be a trusted resource for you to cut through the marketing and health-and-fitness information clutter bombarding you every day. We want to provide you with the best ongoing strategies to upgrade your Mindset, Nutrition, Movement, and Recovery to help build and sustain you for life. We realize that life continually evolves, and we'll be here to offer you solutions and advice. It's a two-way street; we want to hear from and work with you on these solutions.

The platform for this is our website, www.coreperformance.com, which since the publication of *Core Performance* in 2004 has grown into a one-stop resource for performance living, with dozens of respected contributors from the Athletes' Performance and Core Performance communities providing cutting-edge research, tips, and advice to help you thrive in the game of life, all brought into one seamless, individualized system. This site will allow you to truly customize your Core Performance experience, from the moment you wake up to when you go to bed. You can budget how much time you train and on what days, while planning how you will accomplish your loftiest goals. It doesn't matter whether you (or a friend or loved one) have not exercised in years or you are a serious athlete, you will find solutions waiting for you at www.coreperformance.com.

The site is organized into five easy-to-follow categories. Under "Core Knowledge," you'll learn up-to-date ways of training, eating, preparing, and recovering from exercise and the demands of life. It includes recipes and more than five hundred short videos that illustrate the many movements in the Core Performance program, only a fraction of which we were able to include in this book.

Under "Core Daily," you can stay up-to-the-minute with the latest breakthroughs in news and commentary on nutrition, fitness, health, and performance. At a time when newspapers and other media outlets are slashing coverage in this area, we're proud to provide this vital information via articles and blogs written by our accomplished staff of coaches, trainers, nutritionists, and journalists.

Under "Core Talk," you can connect with others who share similar goals and challenges. Whether you're looking to change your life or stick with a plan, it's always easier when you have like-minded people to turn to for support. So visit the forums, engage in lively discussion, find answers, and become part of this world of high-performance social networking.

You might find that the Movement program in this book is enough to sustain you for many years, if not for life. But perhaps you'd like a more customized approach for your specific sport or goal. Under "Training Programs," you'll find countless ways to personalize your plan. It's like having your very own coach, nutritionist, and physical therapist, minus the hefty price tag.

At the Core Store, we provide dozens of products, including all of the Core Performance books and DVDs, apparel, and all of the equipment you need to create a mini Core Performance gym in your home. I know you are incredibly busy, and maybe a gym membership is just not feasible, or maybe you have a membership but are never able to use it. A simple Core Performance Center home gym lets you structure Core Performance around *your* life.

Maybe you're thinking, "Sure, that would be great, but I don't have the space for elaborate equipment." The beauty of this is that the equipment is easy to use and compact. It will fit under your bed or in a small corner of a room. Now that you've become a "Spartan woman," I want you to have Spartan training equipment that packs an incredible punch in such a small space.

All of the products you'll find online are tested and used at Athletes' Performance by the top champions in sport. The Core Store also provides educational DVDs, which will expand on the information in this book, giving you additional levels and progressions of exercises.

Ultimately I want you to be members of the Core Performance online community for life, which is why we provide so much free content and have made a membership available for less than the cost of a weekly cup of coffee. This means that for the cost of a personal training session, you will have progressive programs based upon your lifestyle and accomplishments that evolve with you as your goals and needs change.

Perhaps you're someone who wants an even more personalized Core Performance experience. We recently opened the Core Performance Center in Santa Monica,

California, and have plans to bring these cutting-edge performance centers to every major U.S. market. For more information, visit www.coreperformancecenter.com.

I've had great success supporting people in the pursuit of their dreams, from prominent sports figures, business executives, and parents to readers who have reached spectacular goals. What I love most is being able to build these athletes, these achievers, to see them evolve and reach their goals.

I want to hear how this program has transformed your life. Tell me how it has enabled you to meet challenges, overcome pain and injuries, and fulfill your dreams. Tell the entire Core Performance community how taking a proactive approach to life has enabled you to make a difference in the lives of those you care about most.

Please share your stories with us: Write us via the "Contact Us" page on www .coreperformance.com. We'll pick the most inspirational submissions, the ones that touch us the most, and bring those women to the Core Performance Center to train in person with our world-class staff.

Since we can't bring everyone out, I hope you'll join our online community and interact with the growing number of people dedicated to treating each day as an athletic event and properly preparing themselves for the competition that is the game of life.

You now have the resources to achieve your goals. We've done our part and we will continue to be there for you every day at www.coreperformance.com. I expect you to hold up your end of the relationship and move toward your goals on a daily basis. All of us here in the Core Performance community are honored to be supporting you.

Your coach,
Mark Verstegen

APPENDIX:
THE CORE PERFORMANCE WOMEN
WORKOUT AT A GLANCE

Strength Day Workouts: Level 1

PILLAR PREP

STAGE	A	B	C	D
Sets	1	2	2	2
Reps	6	6	8	10

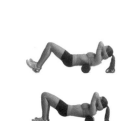

Foam Roll—Thoracic Spine

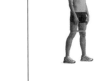

Squat—Mini Band

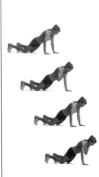

Plank—Kneeling with Shoulder Tap

MOVEMENT PREP

STAGE	A	B	C	D
Sets	1	2	2	2
Reps	4	4	5	6

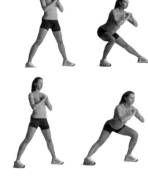

Lateral Squat

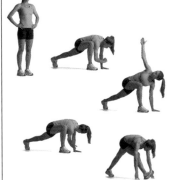

Forward Lunge, Elbow to
Instep + Rotation (in place)

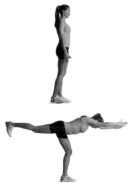

Inverted Hamstring with Reach

STRENGTH/POWER

STAGE	A	B	C	D
Sets	2	2	3	3
Reps	8	10	10	12

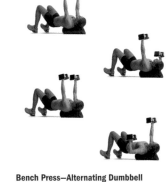

Bench Press—Alternating Dumbbell
(with foam roll)

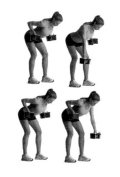

Bent-Over Row—1 Arm, 1 Leg Dumbbell

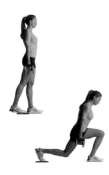

Reverse Lunge—Dumbbell (slide)

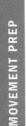
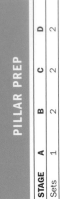
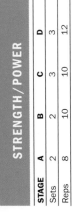
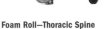

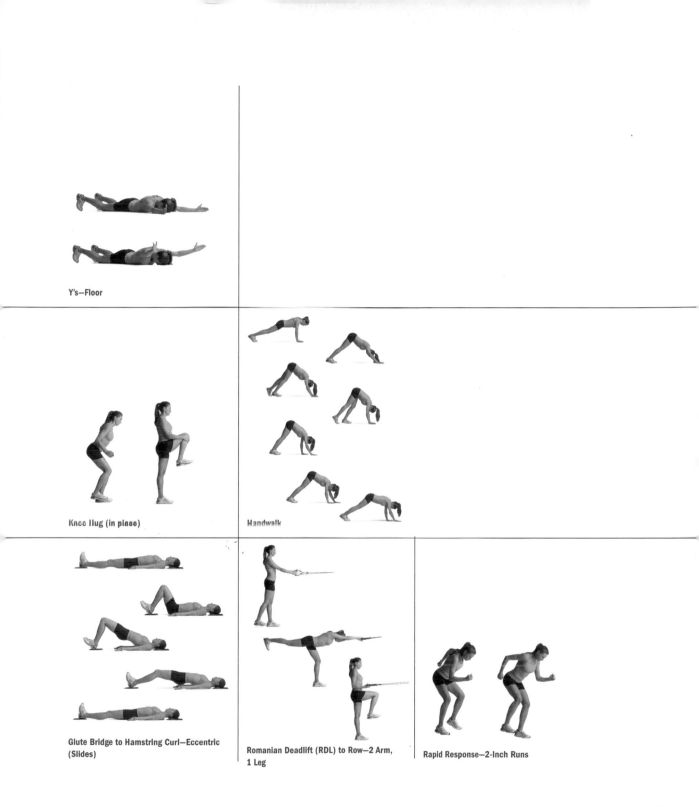

Y's—Floor

Knee Hug (in place)

Handwalk

Glute Bridge to Hamstring Curl—Eccentric
(Slides)

Romanian Deadlift (RDL) to Row—2 Arm,
1 Leg

Rapid Response—2-Inch Runs

Strength Day Workouts: Level 2

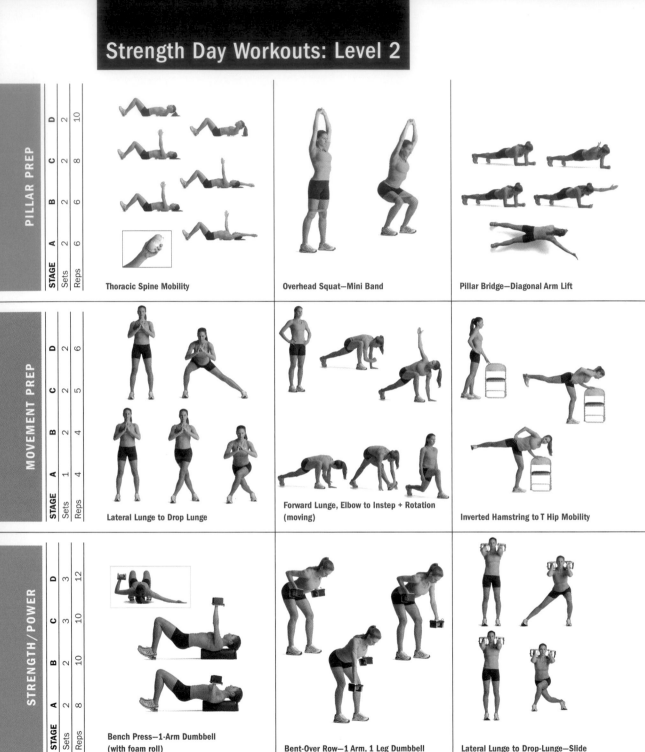

PILLAR PREP

STAGE	A	B	C	D
Sets	2	2	2	2
Reps	6	6	8	10

Thoracic Spine Mobility

Overhead Squat—Mini Band

Pillar Bridge—Diagonal Arm Lift

MOVEMENT PREP

STAGE	A	B	C	D
Sets	1	2	2	2
Reps	4	4	5	6

Lateral Lunge to Drop Lunge

Forward Lunge, Elbow to Instep + Rotation (moving)

Inverted Hamstring to T Hip Mobility

STRENGTH/POWER

STAGE	A	B	C	D
Sets	2	2	3	3
Reps	8	10	10	12

Bench Press—1-Arm Dumbbell (with foam roll)

Bent-Over Row—1 Arm, 1 Leg Dumbbell

Lateral Lunge to Drop-Lunge—Slide

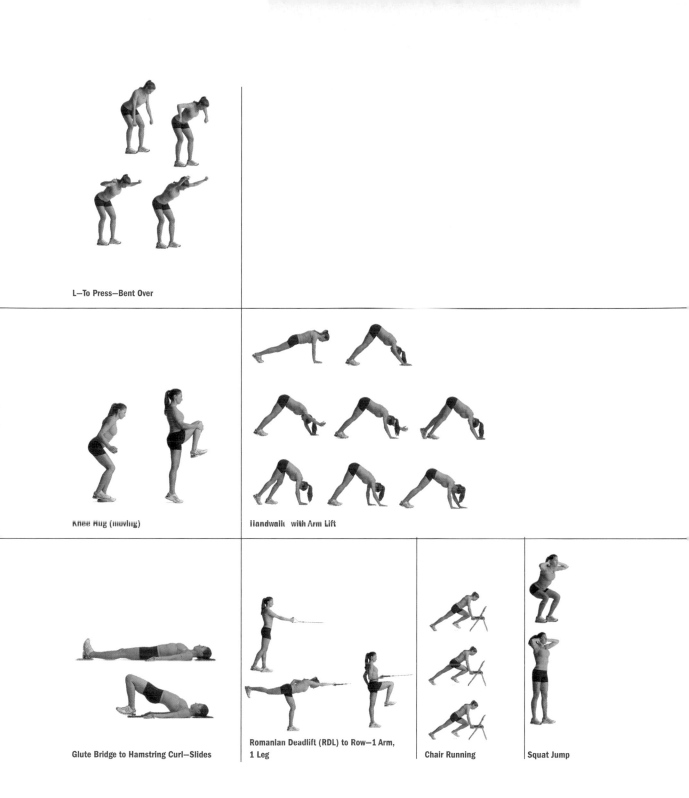

L—To Press—Bent Over

Knee Hug (moving)

Handwalk with Arm Lift

Glute Bridge to Hamstring Curl—Slides

Romanian Deadlift (RDL) to Row—1 Arm, 1 Leg

Chair Running

Squat Jump

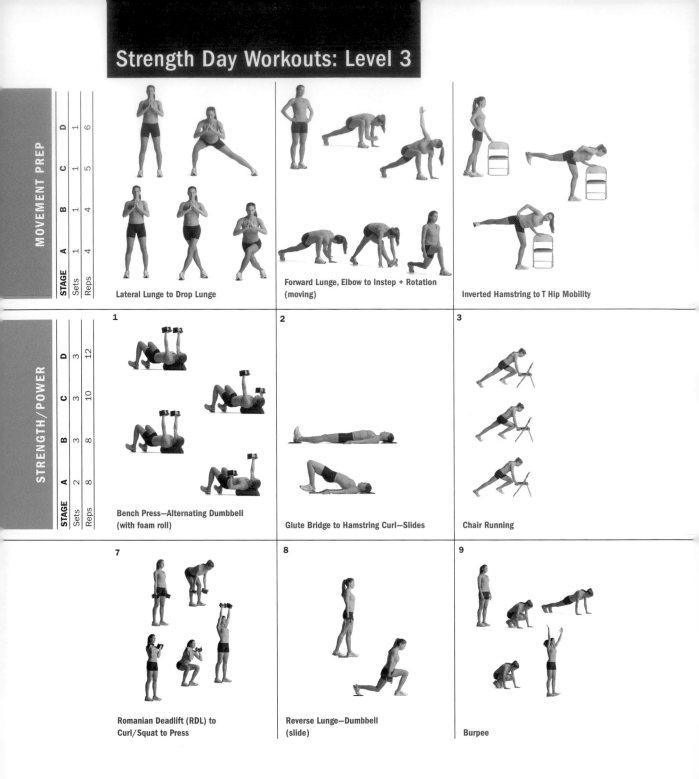

Strength Day Workouts: Level 3

MOVEMENT PREP

STAGE	A	B	C	D
Sets	1	1	1	1
Reps	4	4	5	6

Lateral Lunge to Drop Lunge

Forward Lunge, Elbow to Instep + Rotation (moving)

Inverted Hamstring to T Hip Mobility

STRENGTH/POWER

STAGE	A	B	C	D
Sets	2	3	3	3
Reps	8	8	10	12

1

Bench Press—Alternating Dumbbell (with foam roll)

2

Glute Bridge to Hamstring Curl—Slides

3

Chair Running

7

Romanian Deadlift (RDL) to Curl/Squat to Press

8

Reverse Lunge—Dumbbell (slide)

9

Burpee

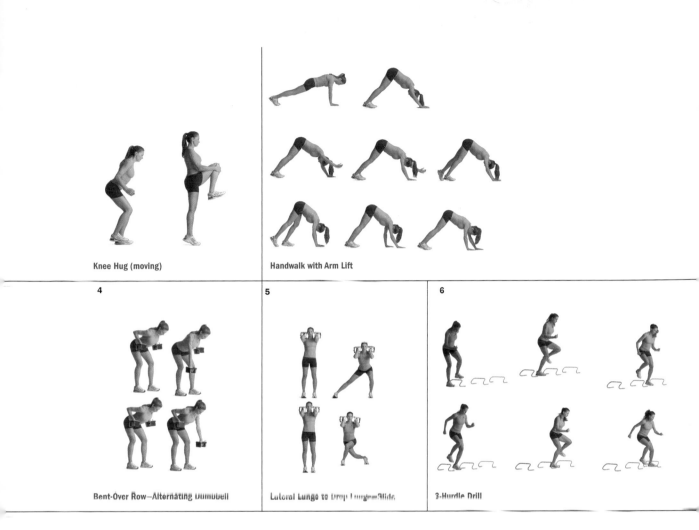

Knee Hug (moving)

Handwalk with Arm Lift

4

Bent-Over Row—Alternating Dumbbell

5

Lateral Lunge to Drop Lunge—Slide

6

3-Hurdle Drill

Endurance Day Workouts: Level 1

PILLAR PREP

STAGE	A	B	C	D
Sets	1	2	2	2
Reps	6	6	8	10

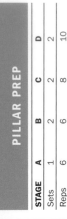
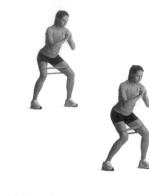

Mini Band External Rotation

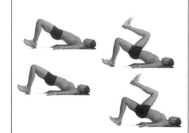

Glute Bridge—Marching Hip Flexion

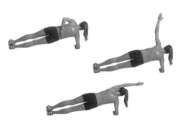

Lateral Pillar Bridge with Pec Stretch

MOVEMENT PREP

STAGE	A	B	C	D
Sets	1	2	2	2
Reps	4	4	5	6

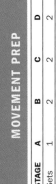
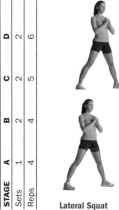
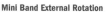

Lateral Squat

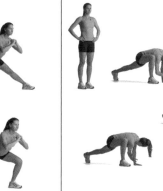

Forward Lunge, Elbow to Instep + Rotation (in place)

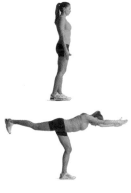

Inverted Hamstring with Reach

ENERGY SYSTEM

STAGE: A

# OF CIRCUITS	TIME	INTENSITY	REPS
1	3 minutes	4 to 5	1
3	3 minutes	7	1
	3 minutes	4 to 5	1

STAGE: B

# OF CIRCUITS	TIME	INTENSITY	REPS
1	3 minutes	4 to 5	1
3	4 minutes	7	1
	2 minutes	4 to 5	1

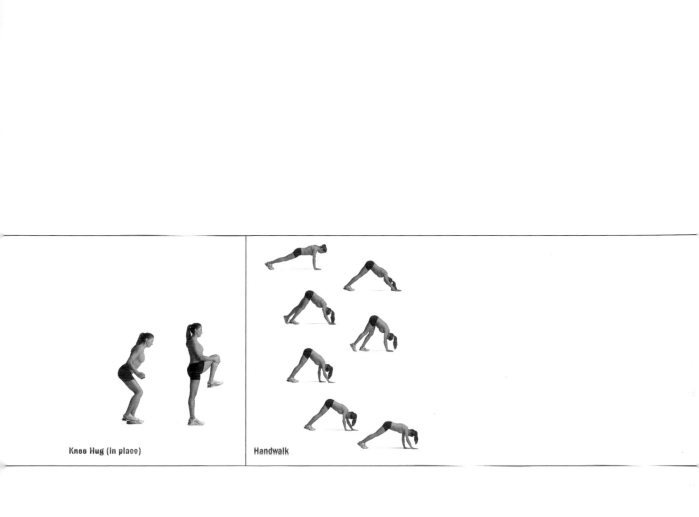

Knee Hug (in place)

Handwalk

STAGE: C

# OF CIRCUITS	TIME	INTENSITY	REPS
1	3 minutes	4 to 5	1
3	5 minutes	7	1
	1 minute	4 to 5	1

STAGE: D

# OF CIRCUITS	TIME	INTENSITY	REPS
1	3 minutes	4 to 5	1
3	30 seconds	8 to 9	1
	2.5 minutes	7	1
	3 minutes	4 to 5	1

Endurance Day Workouts: Level 2

PILLAR PREP

STAGE	A	B	C	D
Sets	2	2	2	2
Reps	6	6	8	10

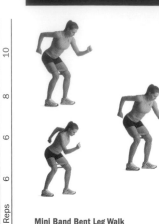

Mini Band Bent Leg Walk

Glute Bridge—Knee Extension with Adduction

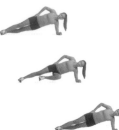

Lateral Pillar Bridge—Marching

MOVEMENT PREP

STAGE	A	B	C	D
Sets	1	1	1	1
Reps	4	4	5	6

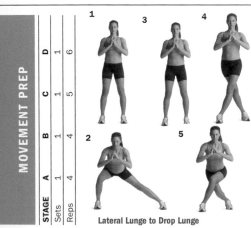

Lateral Lunge to Drop Lunge

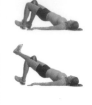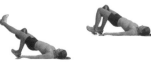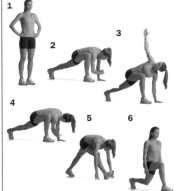

Forward Lunge, Elbow to Instep + Rotation (moving)

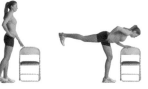

Inverted Hamstring to T Hip Mobility

ENERGY SYSTEM

STAGE: A

# OF CIRCUITS	TIME	INTENSITY	REPS
1	3 minutes	4 to 5	1
4	30 seconds	8 to 9	1
	30 seconds	4 to 5	1
	30 seconds	8 to 9	1
	30 seconds	4 to 5	1
	30 seconds	8 to 9	1
	2.5 minutes	4 to 5	1

STAGE: B

# OF CIRCUITS	TIME	INTENSITY	REPS
1	3 minutes	4 to 5	1
4	30 seconds	8 to 9	1
	30 seconds	4 to 5	1
	30 seconds	8 to 9	1
	30 seconds	4 to 5	1
	30 seconds	8 to 9	1
	2.5 minutes	4 to 5	1

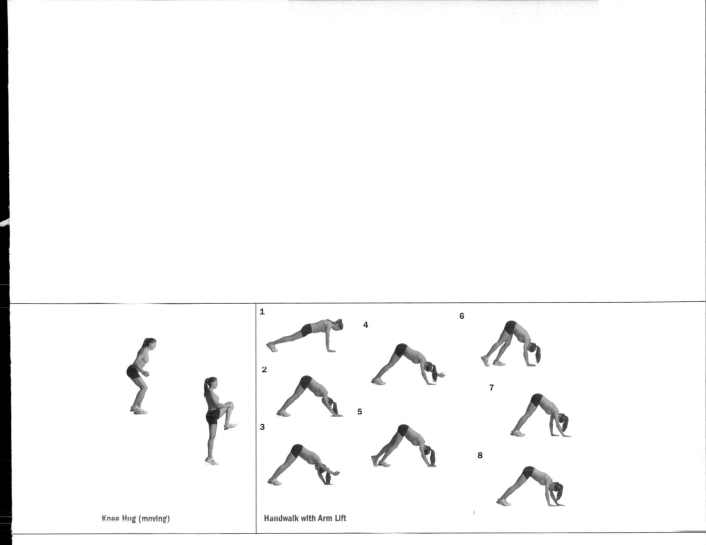

Knee Hug (moving)

Handwalk with Arm Lift

STAGE: C

# OF CIRCUITS	TIME	INTENSITY	REPS
1	2 minutes	4 to 5	1
3	1 minute	8 to 9	1
	1 minute	4 to 5	1
	1 minute	8 to 9	1
	1 minute	4 to 5	1
	1 minute	8 to 9	1
	2 minutes	4 to 5	1

STAGE: D

# OF CIRCUITS	TIME	INTENSITY	REPS
1	3 minutes	4 to 5	1
2	1 minute	8 to 9	1
	1 minute	4 to 5	1
	1 minute	8 to 9	1
	1 minute	4 to 5	1
	1 minute	8 to 9	1
	1 minute	4 to 5	1
	1 minute	8 to 9	1
	3 minutes	4 to 5	1

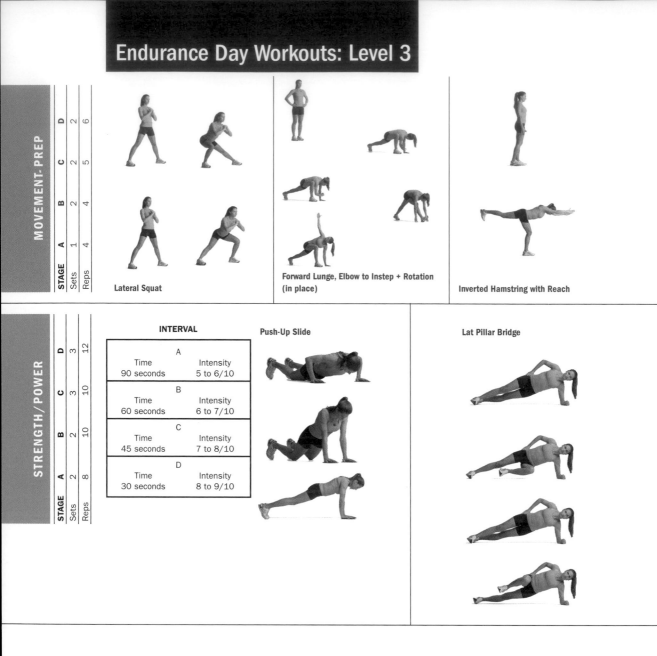

Endurance Day Workouts: Level 3

MOVEMENT- PREP

STAGE	A	B	C	D
Sets	1	2	2	2
Reps	4	4	5	6

Lateral Squat

Forward Lunge, Elbow to Instep + Rotation (in place)

Inverted Hamstring with Reach

STRENGTH/POWER

STAGE	A	B	C	D
Sets	2	2	3	3
Reps	8	10	10	12

INTERVAL

	A	
Time	Intensity	
90 seconds	5 to 6/10	

	B	
Time	Intensity	
60 seconds	6 to 7/10	

	C	
Time	Intensity	
45 seconds	7 to 8/10	

	D	
Time	Intensity	
30 seconds	8 to 9/10	

Push-Up Slide

Lat Pillar Bridge

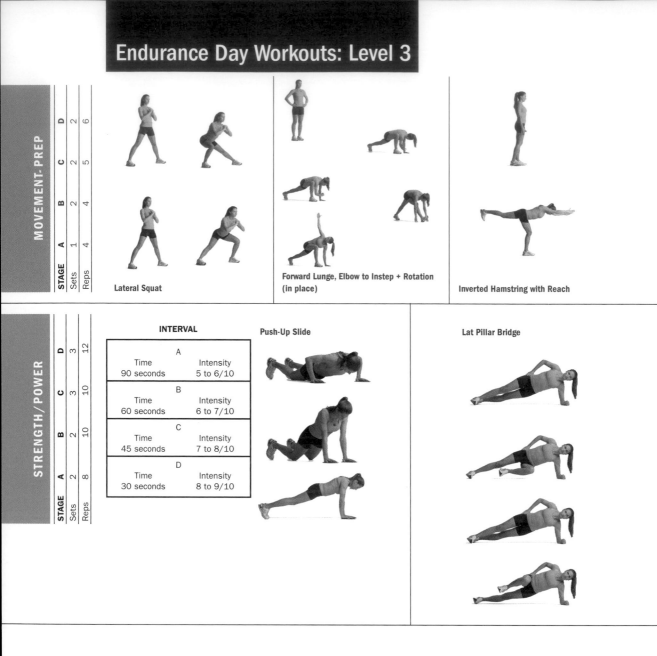

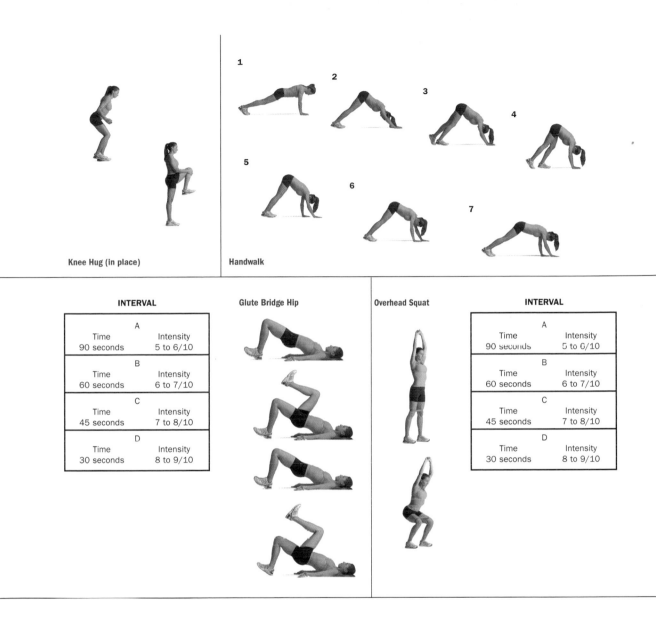

Knee Hug (in place)

Handwalk

1
2
3
4
5
6
7

INTERVAL

	A	
Time		Intensity
90 seconds		5 to 6/10

	B	
Time		Intensity
60 seconds		6 to 7/10

	C	
Time		Intensity
45 seconds		7 to 8/10

	D	
Time		Intensity
30 seconds		8 to 9/10

Glute Bridge Hip

Overhead Squat

INTERVAL

	A	
Time		Intensity
90 seconds		5 to 6/10

	B	
Time		Intensity
60 seconds		6 to 7/10

	C	
Time		Intensity
45 seconds		7 to 8/10

	D	
Time		Intensity
30 seconds		8 to 9/10

1. Thoracic Spine Mobility

2. Trigger Point—Glute

3. Trigger Point—
TFL (Tensor Fasciae Latae)

4. Trigger Point—Neck

9. Foam Roll—
TFL (Tensor Fasciae Latae)

10. Foam Roll—IT (Iliotibial) Band

11. Reach, Roll—Foam Roll

12. AIS Kneeling Quad/Hip Flexor

5. Foam Roll—Glute

6. Foam Roll—Lower Back and QL (Quadratus Lumborum)

7. Foam Roll—Thoracic Spine

8. Foam Roll—Quad/Hip Flexor

13. AIS Kneeling Adductor

14. AIS Bent-Knee Hamstring

15. AIS Abductor

16. AIS Side-Lying Shoulder Stretch

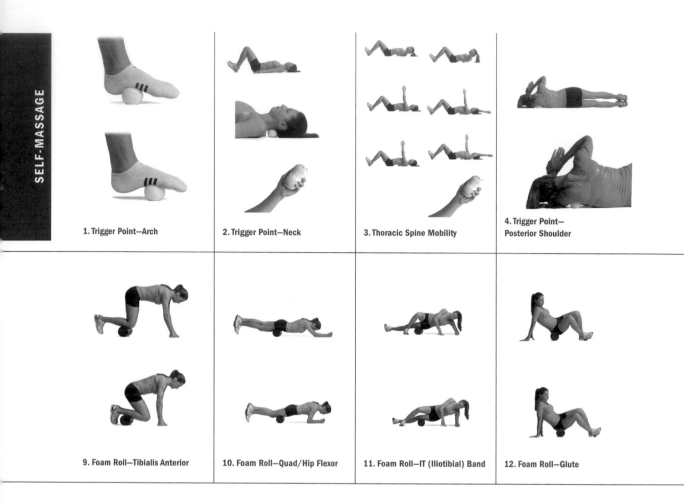

1. Trigger Point—Arch

2. Trigger Point—Neck

3. Thoracic Spine Mobility

4. Trigger Point—Posterior Shoulder

9. Foam Roll—Tibialis Anterior

10. Foam Roll—Quad/Hip Flexor

11. Foam Roll—IT (Iliotibial) Band

12. Foam Roll—Glute

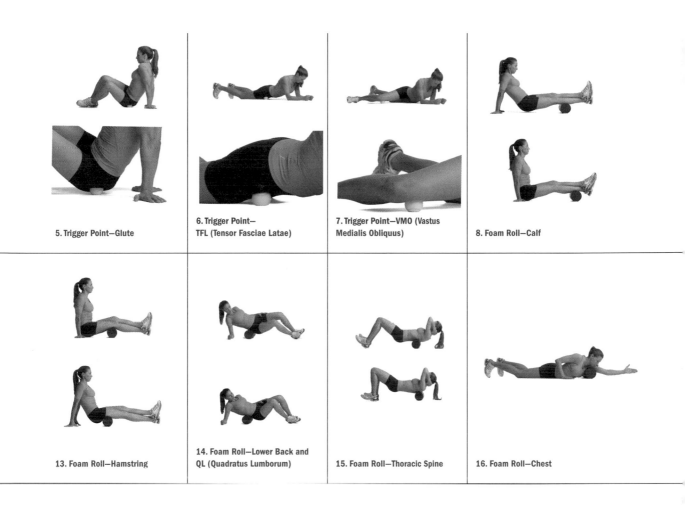

5. Trigger Point—Glute

6. Trigger Point— TFL (Tensor Fasciae Latae)

7. Trigger Point—VMO (Vastus Medialis Obliquus)

8. Foam Roll—Calf

13. Foam Roll—Hamstring

14. Foam Roll—Lower Back and QL (Quadratus Lumborum)

15. Foam Roll—Thoracic Spine

16. Foam Roll—Chest

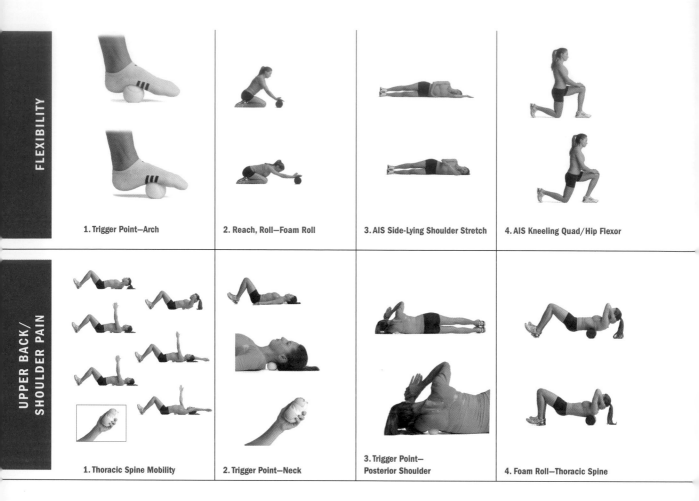

FLEXIBILITY

1. Trigger Point—Arch

2. Reach, Roll—Foam Roll

3. AIS Side-Lying Shoulder Stretch

4. AIS Kneeling Quad/Hip Flexor

UPPER BACK/ SHOULDER PAIN

1. Thoracic Spine Mobility

2. Trigger Point—Neck

3. Trigger Point— Posterior Shoulder

4. Foam Roll—Thoracic Spine

5. AIS Kneeling Adductor

6. AIS Bent-Knee Hamstring

7. AIS Abductor

5. Foam Roll—Chest

6. Foam Roll—Lower Back and QL (Quadratus Lumborum)

7. Reach, Roll Foam Roll

8. AIS—Side-Lying Shoulder Stretch

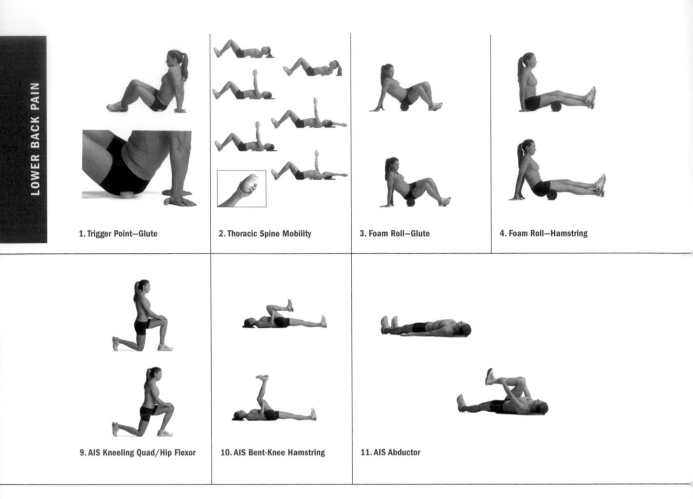

LOWER BACK PAIN

1. Trigger Point—Glute

2. Thoracic Spine Mobility

3. Foam Roll—Glute

4. Foam Roll—Hamstring

9. AIS Kneeling Quad/Hip Flexor

10. AIS Bent-Knee Hamstring

11. AIS Abductor

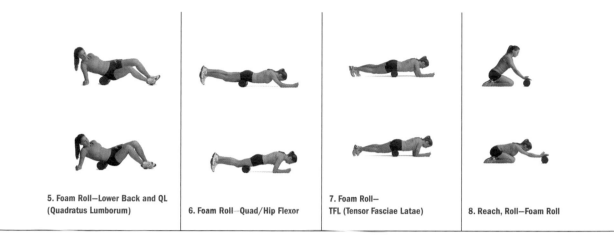

5. Foam Roll—Lower Back and QL (Quadratus Lumborum)

6. Foam Roll—Quad/Hip Flexor

7. Foam Roll— TFL (Tensor Fasciae Latae)

8. Reach, Roll—Foam Roll

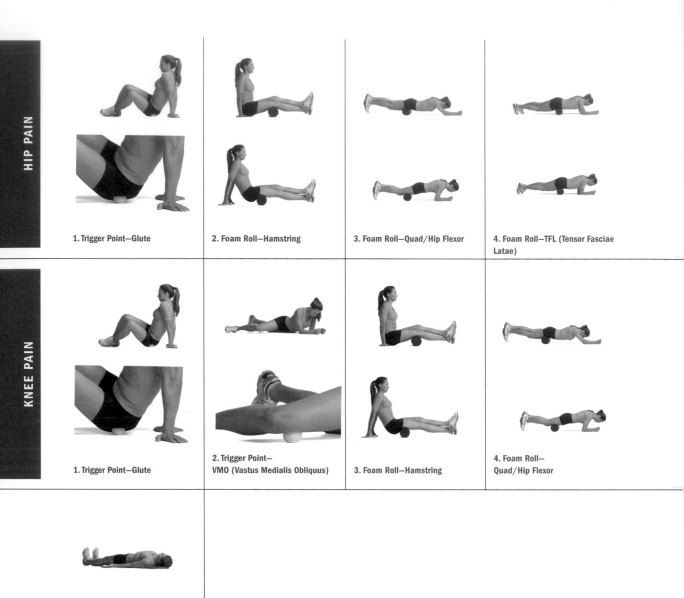

HIP PAIN

1. Trigger Point—Glute

2. Foam Roll—Hamstring

3. Foam Roll—Quad/Hip Flexor

4. Foam Roll—TFL (Tensor Fasciae Latae)

KNEE PAIN

1. Trigger Point—Glute

2. Trigger Point—VMO (Vastus Medialis Obliquus)

3. Foam Roll—Hamstring

4. Foam Roll—Quad/Hip Flexor

9. AIS Abductor

5. Foam Roll—IT (Iliotibial) Band

6. AIS Bent-Knee Hamstring

7. AIS Kneeling Quad/Hip Flexor

8. AIS—Kneeling Adductor

5. Foam Roll—
TFL (Tensor Fasciae Latae)

6. Foam Roll—
IT (Iliotibial) Band

7. AIS Bent-Knee Hamstring

8. AIS Kneeling Quad/Hip Flexor

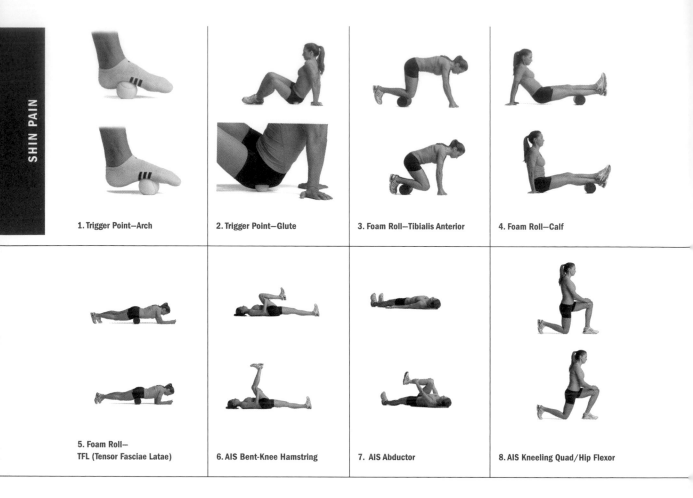

1. Trigger Point—Arch

2. Trigger Point—Glute

3. Foam Roll—Tibialis Anterior

4. Foam Roll—Calf

5. Foam Roll—
TFL (Tensor Fasciae Latae)

6. AIS Bent-Knee Hamstring

7. AIS Abductor

8. AIS Kneeling Quad/Hip Flexor

FAQS

Q: When is the best time to train?

A: Whenever it fits into your schedule. Many people prefer first thing in the morning, even if that means getting up an hour early. It's a great way to jump-start your day and gives you a feeling of accomplishment from the get-go. You don't have to worry about your workout time being compromised by something unforeseen at work or at home. Women in the corporate world might find it easier to train during lunch break or immediately after work. Stay-at-home moms might find it preferable to work out in the mid to late morning, after the kids have left for school. Women in high school and college might prefer the afternoons, immediately after class. The key is to schedule training on your planner, preferably at a consistent time, and book it in your daily calendar.

Q: Why won't I get bulky doing strength training in the Core Performance system?

A: I hear this a lot: "I don't want to lift weights because it will make me bulky." If you train with methods designed to train you like a bodybuilder, you might lean that way, at least in theory, but women don't have the male hormones necessary to get big. Women who are bulking up are using chemicals that you want no part of. With the Core Performance system, you'll better lengthen and strengthen your muscles, giving your body much more fluid motion and a much more fluid look.

Q: Will I lose weight or gain weight with this program?

A: The key is to stop using the scale as the scorecard. Measure yourself by appearance, not by the scale. Weight is weight. A pound of muscle is equal to a pound of fat on the scale. By girth and by measurement, they're two totally different things. A pound of muscle might look like a couple of pencils tied together, but a pound of fat might look like one or two softballs wrapped together. The scale will tell you they're the same. Two 135-pound women could look dramatically different. The Core Performance system is going to help you lose body fat but also maintain or slightly increase lean body mass, which ultimately will keep you lean and fit throughout your life span.

Q: I do a lot of cardio. Isn't that enough?

A: No, and the reason for that is we're trying to make positive change, and that takes a world-class system, not just one finite tool where you're trying to make different things out of the same stimulus. How many people do you see who go to the gym all the time but their bodies never change? They're doing the same thing day in and day out and expecting a different result, but the body does not work that way. Our goal is to create more efficient movement patterns that will produce mobility and stability while lengthening and strengthening muscles, enabling you to make sustainable gains throughout your life. You can continue to improve your strength and energy systems decade after decade.

The problem with being a so-called cardio queen is that you rarely reach the intensity levels you need to make significant change. With our Energy System Development unit, you're going through your different energy systems, stimulating your body to burn body fat, stimulating your lean body mass, and influencing your body's hormones in a positive manner. Best of all, you're going to train in a way where you're not going to do the same stale routines, which can lead to overtraining, plateaus, and frustration.

Q: So how come some people who do a lot of cardio never seem to burn fat?

A: It comes down to strength training and lean body mass. Let's look at the typical female jogger. Her lean body mass is that of a low horsepower four-cylinder engine. At rest and even during exercise she's only going to expend so much energy. And if she doesn't start to boost her lean body mass she's not going to improve her running time. She won't expend more force into the ground or into the pedal or swim stroke. She's not going to burn more calories at rest, which the lean body mass created by strength training helps you accomplish. After the age of thirty, you lose a pound of lean body mass per year. You might lose two or three pounds a year if you aren't doing any kind of resistance training. We want to keep that lean body mass with us so we can sustain a high quality of life even in our later years. Think of this resistance training as making a long-term investment in your quality-of-life portfolio.

Q: How much weight should I lift?

A: Women tend to use weights that are far too light. It gets back to that fear of becoming bulky. Keeping yourself constantly challenged and stimulated is the key to any program.

Intensity is far more important than volume, and if women are only using the five-pound or eight-pound "Barbie weights" because they're worried that they'll get bulky if they lift heavier are wasting their time. Ironically, they're hoisting heavier weights than that in their daily lives, whether in the form of toddlers, backpacks, briefcases, and groceries. We're striving to create efficient movement patterns, and progressing from fifteen pounds to thirty-five pounds on an exercise doesn't necessarily mean those muscles are going to get bigger. It just means those muscles are going to get a lot smarter; the process is as much neurological as it is about the size of the muscle. You're making the muscle more efficient, so don't be scared of using heavier weights. This system is not going to make you big and bulky. If you're only using the lighter weights, it will compromise your results. Pick the heaviest weight you can handle to complete the designated reps.

Q: Is it true women's muscles recover faster than those of men?

A: Under a microscope, there is no difference between male and female tissue, no difference on the cellular level. The hormonal profiles are what are significantly different. The only reason a female would recover faster is if she is in a higher training state and she did a relatively easy workout that placed less stress on her body. If someone did an equal workout and felt like she recovered faster, it's just because she didn't push herself as hard. Muscle cells are muscle cells. Women, like men, can do a better job of implementing a system of nutrition and sleep that facilitates recovery better.

Q: Is dieting harder on women than men?

A: Not necessarily. But because women have less lean body mass than men, the effects of fad and yo-yo diets are more pronounced with women. Most diets are engineered to lose weight. It doesn't matter what the weight is. Ideally it's fat, but more commonly it's water and even lean body mass. When you regain that weight, as you inevitably will on these nonsustainable diets, the weight doesn't come back as lean body mass. That's why it's such a concern when an older person breaks a hip and is bedridden for a period of time. She loses lean mass, strength, and bone mass, and when she's able to get up she's at half of her former capacity and she's never going to get that back. That's ultimately what happens to women of any age on these diets. They're effectively transformed from a four-cylinder engine to a two-cylinder engine, burning no passive calories even at rest. Now most calories they eat are not needed and are ultimately stored as body fat. We want to turn this process around, creating a six-cylinder engine that will burn more calories even at rest.

ACKNOWLEDGMENTS

The cover of this book features the names of two men—as is the case with many things in life, guys take the credit for the inspiration and contributions of women. This is especially true with this book, which would be pretty flimsy were it not for the insight of many women from the Athletes' Performance and Core Performance communities. At the top of the list is Amanda Carlson, the Director of Performance Nutrition at Athletes' Performance, who spearheaded the Nutrition section of this book. A hearty thank you also goes to Sue Falsone, Anna Hartman, Katie Burke, Sarah Snyder, Danielle LaFata, Debbie Martell, and Karen Bedel.

This book would not exist at all were it not for Avery editor Megan Newman, who challenged us to take a successful franchise up a notch and make it especially applicable to this demanding audience.

Two men have shaped the Core Performance books from the beginning. Craig Friedman's title at Athletes' Performance is Director of the Performance Innovation Team, and he once again has assembled the perfect training regimen. If David Black were not the best literary agent in the business, he could work in my field. He is a true performance coach, motivating his clients to levels they never thought possible.

Finally, the two guys listed on the cover would get little done were it not for their better halves. To Amy Verstegen and Suzy Williams, thanks for making it all possible.

ABOUT THE AUTHORS

Mark Verstegen is recognized as one of the world's most innovative sports performance experts. As the owner of Athletes' Performance—cutting-edge training centers in Phoenix, Los Angeles, Dallas, and Gulf Breeze, Florida—he directs teams of performance specialists and nutritionists to train some of the biggest names in sports.

By teaching an integrated lifestyle and training program that blends strength, speed, flexibility, joint and core stability, and mental toughness, Verstegen helps athletes become not only faster and stronger but also more powerful, flexible, and resistant to injury and long-term back, hip, and other joint problems.

Because of his innovative techniques and up-to-date knowledge of sports performance, Verstegen is a sought-after consultant. He serves as Director of Performance for the NFL Players Association, is an advisor to Adidas, EAS, Gatorade, and other leading performance-oriented companies, and serves as a consultant to numerous athletic governing bodies.

Core Performance, Verstegen's consumer performance brand, is a leading interactive community of thousands of high achievers and can be found at www.coreperformance.com. In 2008 Verstegen opened the first Core Performance Center. Located in Santa Monica, California, it is quickly redefining the concepts of health clubs and personal training.

Verstegen is a dynamic speaker and travels the world to address groups such as the American College of Sports Medicine, the National Strength and Conditioning Association, and many corporate audiences.

Verstegen and his training methods have been profiled by hundreds of national media outlets. He has served as contributing columnist to *Men's Health* and *Best Life* magazines, and his first book, *Core Performance*, sparked the core training fitness phenomenon. The success of that book led to three additional titles: *Core Performance Essentials* (2006), *Core Performance Endurance* (2007), and *Core Performance Golf* (2008).

Verstegen began his coaching career at his alma mater, Washington State University. He served as Assistant Director of Player Development at Georgia Tech and in 1994 created the International Performance Institute on the campus of the IMG Sports Academy in Bradenton, Florida. In 1999 he moved to Phoenix to build Athletes' Performance, which quickly became the industry leader for training world-class athletes.

Verstegen and his wife, Amy, live in Scottsdale, Arizona.

Pete Williams has written about fitness, business, and sports for numerous publications, including *USA Today, The New York Times, Men's Health,* and *SportsBusiness Journal.* He is author or coauthor of eleven books, including the four previous *Core Performance* titles (with Mark Verstegen), *Fun Is Good* (with Mike Veeck), and *The Draft: A Year inside the NFL's Search for Talent.* A graduate of the University of Virginia, an avid triathlete, and a popular keynote speaker, Williams lives in Safety Harbor, Florida, with his wife, Suzy, and their two sons. He hosts the *Fitness Buff* radio show on BlogTalk Radio. His website address is www.petewilliams.net.